Copyright © 2025 by Satisha Monroe

All rights reserved. No part of this publication may be reproduced, stored in a retrieval system, or transmitted in any form or by any means electronic, mechanical, photocopying, recording, or otherwise without the prior written permission of the author.

ISBN: **979-8-218-84866-8**

Printed in the United States of America.

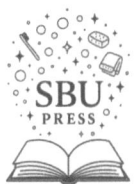

AUTHOR'S NOTE

This book was born from something deeply personal; a legacy of love and cleanliness passed down by my grandmother. Gran made sure every one of us: her children, grandchildren, and great-grandchildren knew how to care for our bodies and understood that hygiene matters. She taught us with patience, consistency, and pride.

Not everyone was given that kind of guidance. There are people, children, teens, even adults who were never taught how to care for their bodies properly. Many have shared painful memories of being sent to school in dirty clothes and teased relentlessly. It wasn't because they didn't care, or because they were just "slobs". In many cases, those responsible for them simply didn't have the knowledge, the capacity, or means to teach them. Some may have been struggling themselves, with mental health, their own unhealed past or just basic survival. Whatever the reason, the result was the same: a child left to feel ashamed of something they were never given the tools to fix.

This book is for anyone who never got that chance. It's for kids, for parents, for people with special needs, and for anyone who needs a reset. If you were never taught how to care for yourself, it's not your fault. But now, we're here to help. You can learn. You can teach others. You can break the cycle! Not only did Sudsy and I make this for you, but so did Gran. Her love, her lessons, and her legacy live in every single page. She didn't know that what she taught us, with all her patience, pride, and consistency, would one day reach the world. But it has. Gran said, "I taught them all how to wash themselves," and she did. Through these pages, she's teaching you too! This book is proof. Now the whole world will know her name.

Thank you, Bessie May Pugh.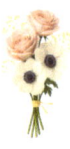

Sincerely,
Satisha Monroe

"Well, I taught them all how to wash themselves."

—Gran ♥

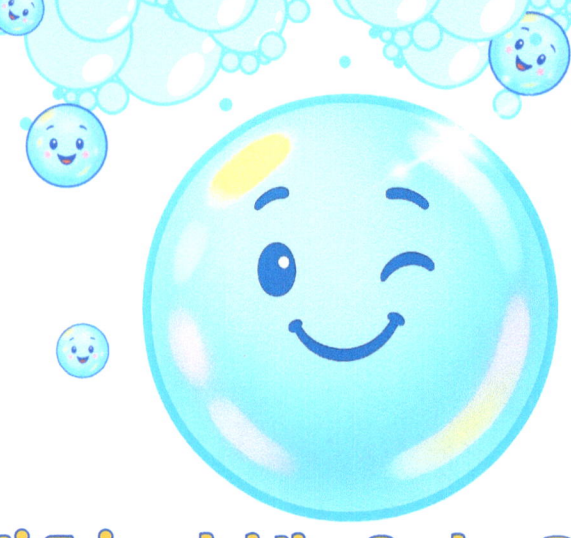

Hi Friends! I'm Sudsy Bubble!

I'M SO GLAD TO SEE YOU AND CAN'T WAIT TO TEACH YOU ALL ABOUT HYGIENE! WHAT'S HYGIENE? IT'S HOW WE KEEP OURSELVES NICE AND CLEAN WITH THINGS LIKE:

SOAP AND WATER, BODYWASH, SHAMPOO, TOOTHPASTE AND WIPES!

IT'S WASHING OUR HANDS WHEN THEY GET ICKY AND SCRUBBING OUR TOES SO THEY DON'T GET STINKY. BUT THOSE GERMIES CAN GET A BIT TRICKY YOU SEE, SO I CALL IN MY LITTLE COUSINS, THE BUBBIES TO SCRUB WITH ME!

IN THIS BOOK YOU'LL LEARN:
- BATH VS SHOWER.
- SPOTS AND STEPS WE FORGET.
- HOW OFTEN TO WASH.
- WHERE AND HOW TO WASH.
- HOW TO CARE FOR YOUR TOWELS.
- HOW TO CARE FOR YOUR MIND AND HEART!

YOU'LL SEE US FLOATING THROUGH THESE PAGES, WITH PICTURES AND WORDS TELLING YOU EXACTLY WHAT TO DO, AND WHEN YOU SEE THOSE BEAUTIFUL POPS OF COLOR, THAT MEANS COME COLOR WITH US TOO!

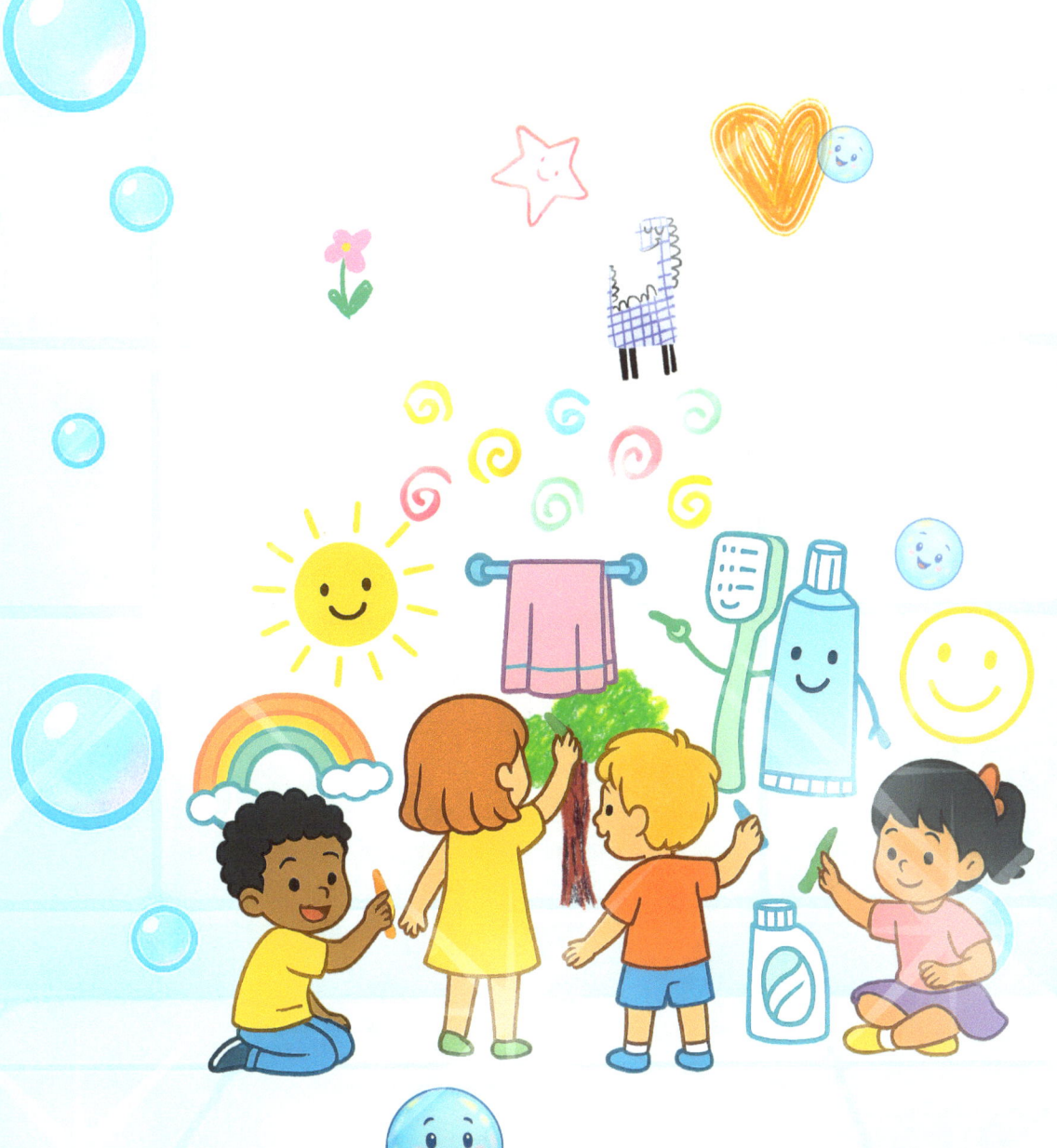

REMEMBER!
EVERYONE'S BODY IS DIFFERENT. IF YOUR HEALTH NEEDS ARE UNIQUE, THAT'S OKAY! YOU CAN STILL LEARN AND COLOR WITH US!

Meet My Germies and Bubbies.

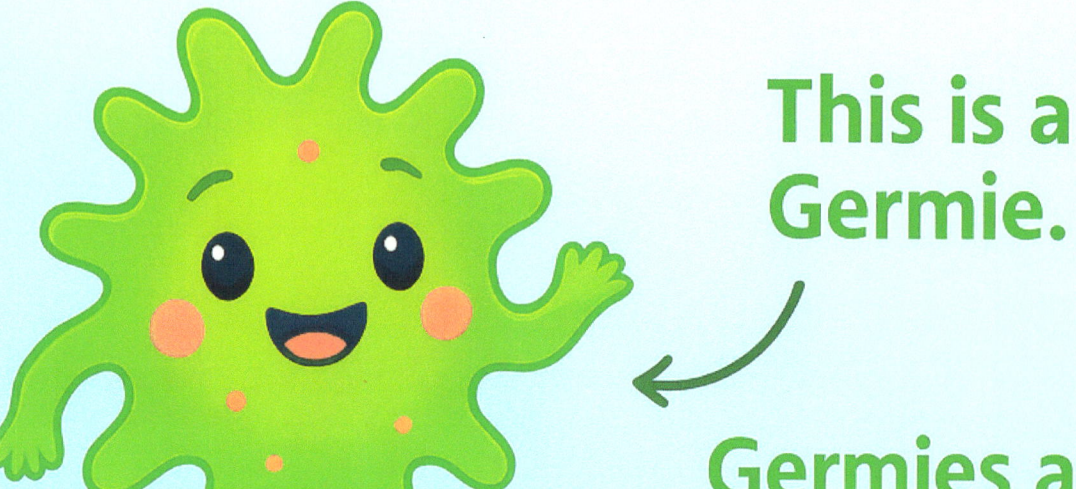

This is a Germie.

Germies are tiny little bacteria that can make us stinky or sick.

...and this is a Bubby.

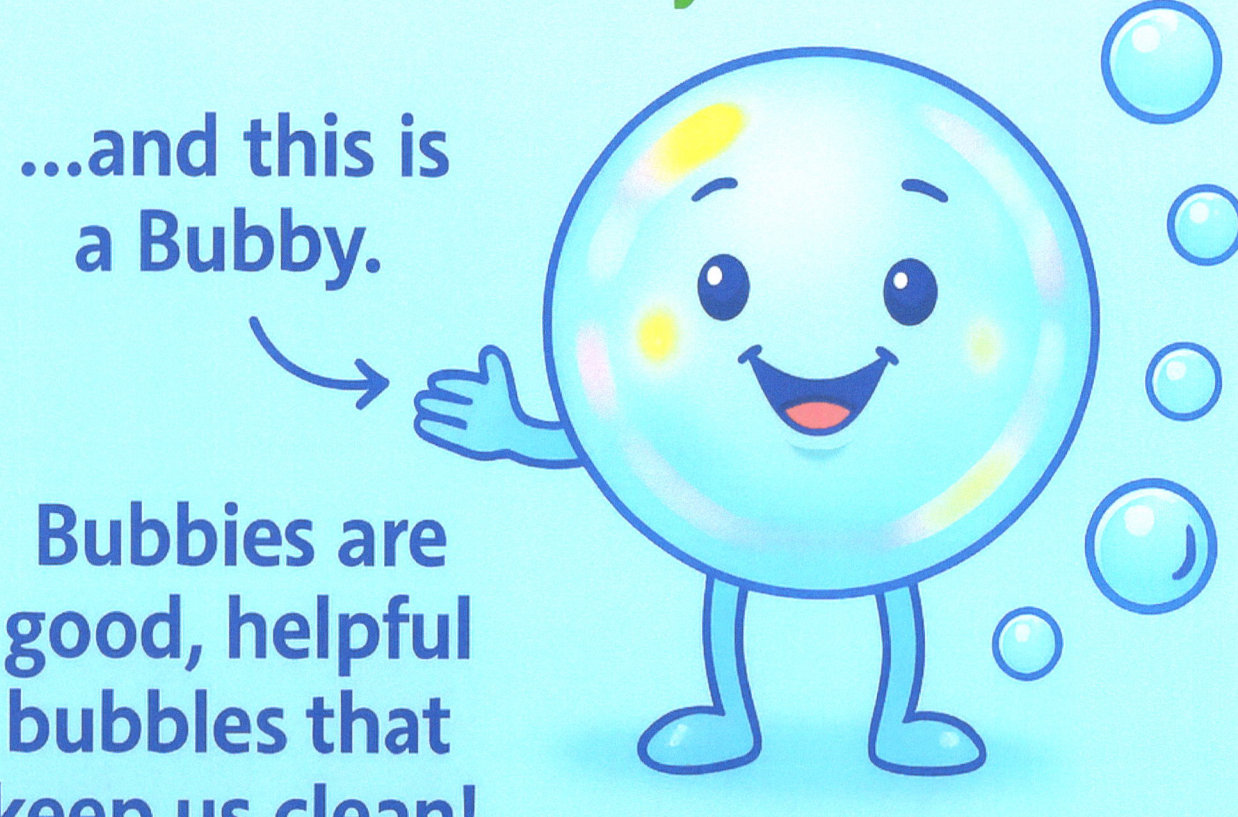

Bubbies are good, helpful bubbles that keep us clean!

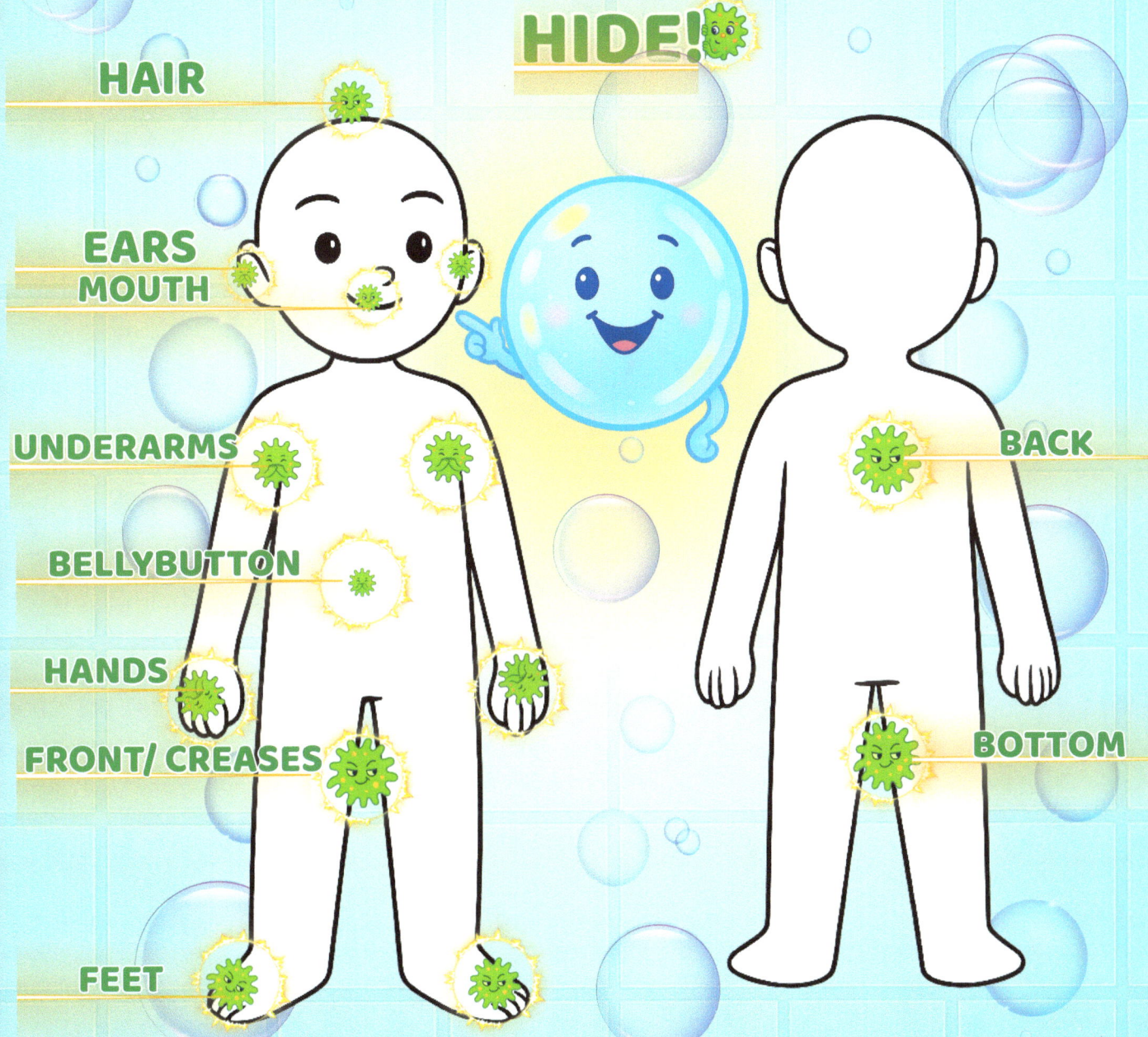

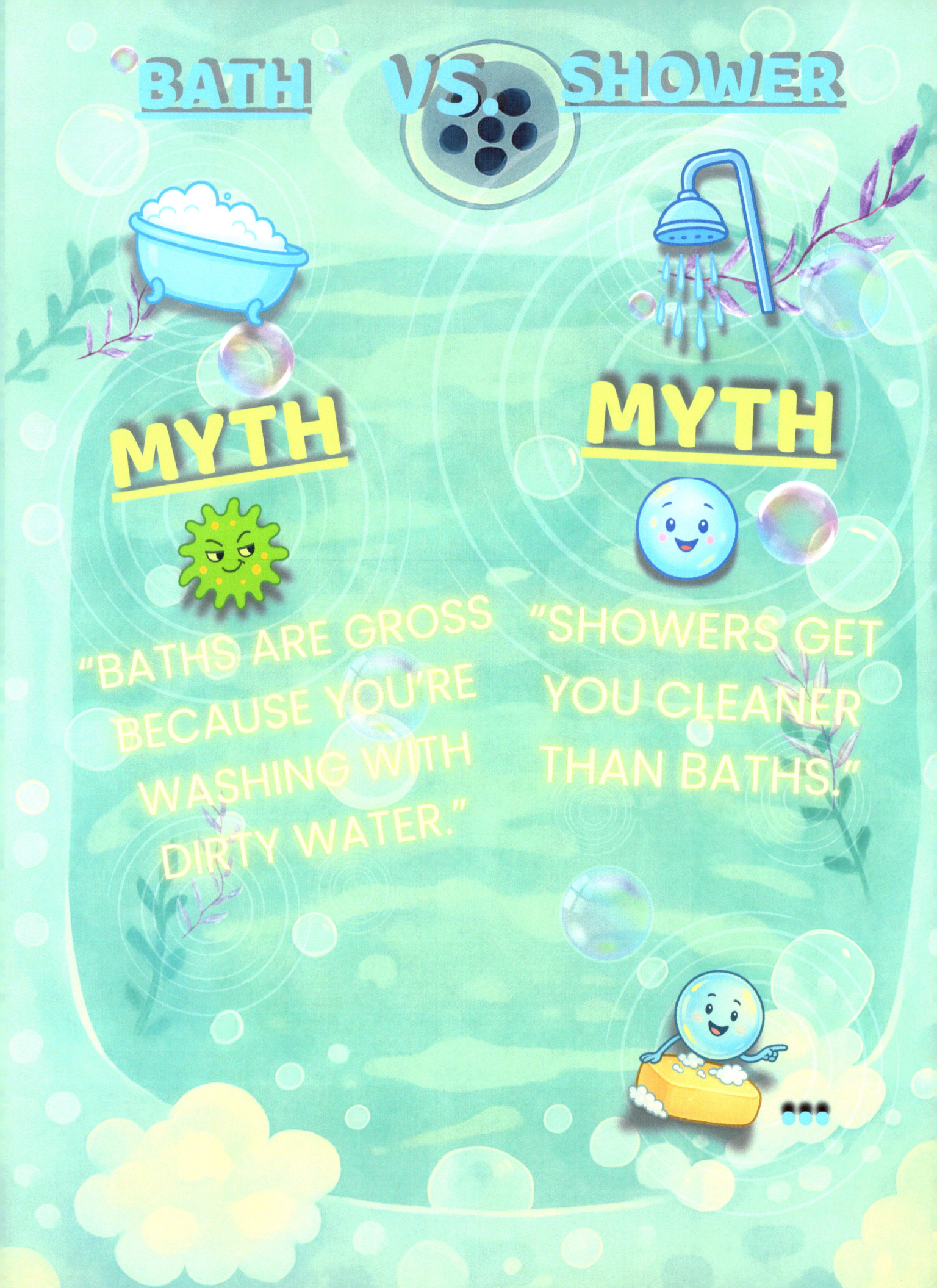

BATH VS. SHOWER

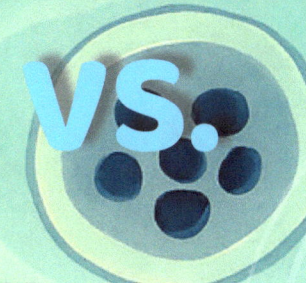

THE TRUTH

1. WHEN YOU LATHER WITH SOAP, THE SOAP GRABS ONTO DIRT, OILS, AND GERMIES, THIS IS CALLED EMULSIFICATION. IT LETS THE DIRT, OIL AND GERMIES LIFT OFF YOUR SKIN AND FLOAT IN THE WATER INSTEAD OF STICKING TO YOU.

2. GERMIES GET SPREAD OUT THROUGH ALL THE BATH WATER, SO THEY BECOME LESS STRONG AND LESS CONCENTRATED, THIS IS CALLED DILUTION.

3. THERE IS SOMETHING LIKE A SOFT, INVISIBLE SKIN ON TOP OF THE WATER THAT HELPS KEEP THE FLOATING DIRT AND GERMIES PUSHED AWAY FROM YOU. THIS IS CALLED SURFACE TENSION. IT'S WHY YOU MIGHT SEE A RING OF DIRT FLOATING AROUND THE EDGE OF THE TUB INSTEAD OF ON YOU. WHEN YOU STEP OUT OF THE TUB, YOU LEAVE ALL THE YUCKY STUFF BEHIND! ALL CLEAN!

THE TRUTH

1. SHOWERS LET YOU WASH YOUR BODY WITH RUNNING WATER.

2. WHEN YOU LATHER WITH SOAP, THE SOAP GRABS ONTO DIRT, OILS, AND GERMIES, THIS IS CALLED EMULSIFICATION. IT LETS DIRT, OILS AND GERMIES LIFT OFF YOUR SKIN AND FLOW DOWN THE DRAIN.

3. WHEN YOU STEP OUT OF THE SHOWER, YOU ARE ALL CLEAN!

SUDSY TIP!

ALWAYS:
- START WITH A CLEAN TUB.
- IF HAVING A BATH, RUN FRESH WATER.
- **NEVER** SHARE BATH WATER!
- CLEAN TUB WHEN DONE.

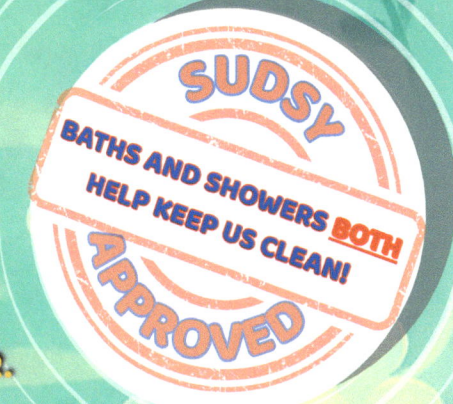

SUDSY APPROVED — BATHS AND SHOWERS **BOTH** HELP KEEP US CLEAN!

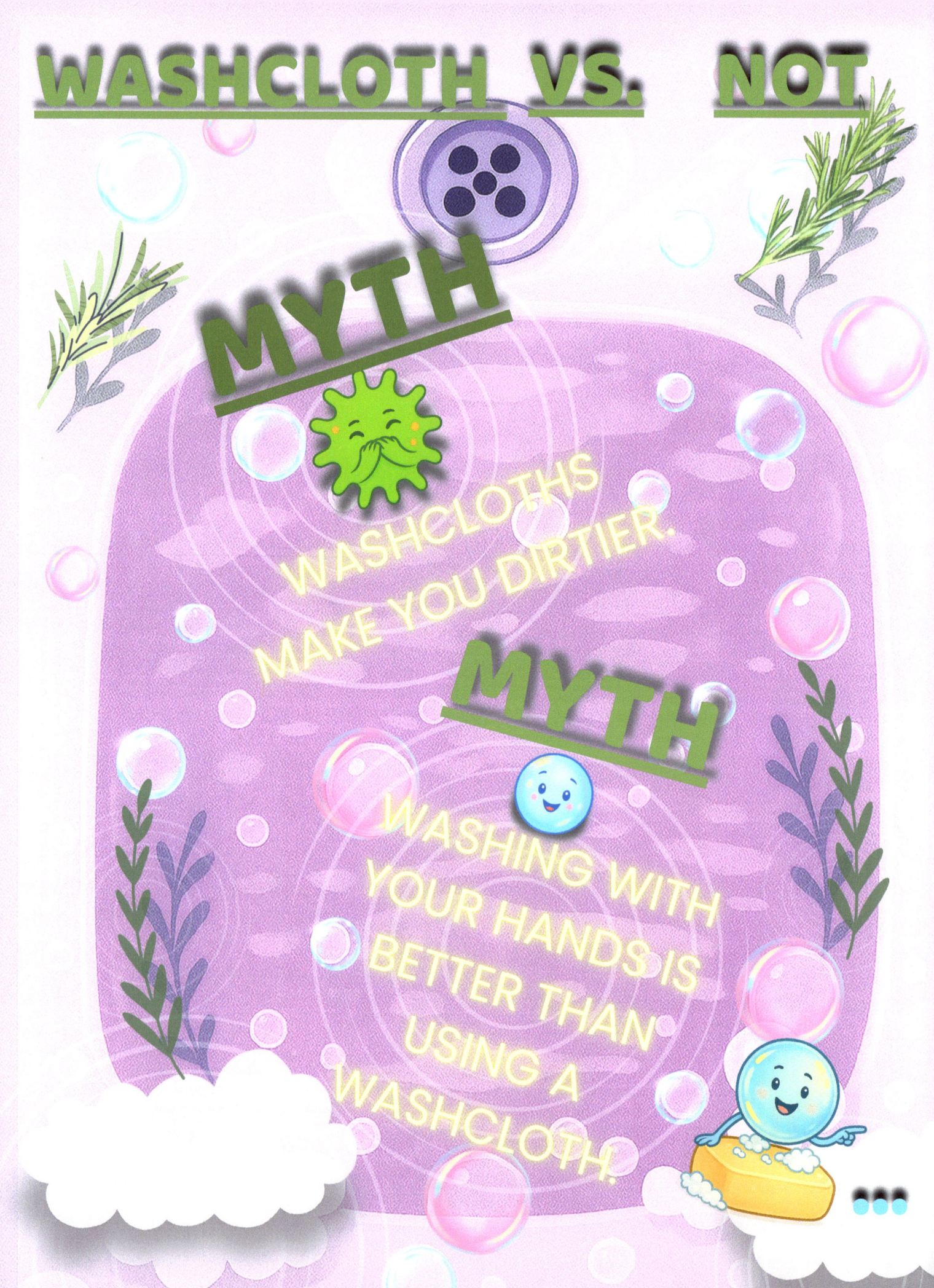

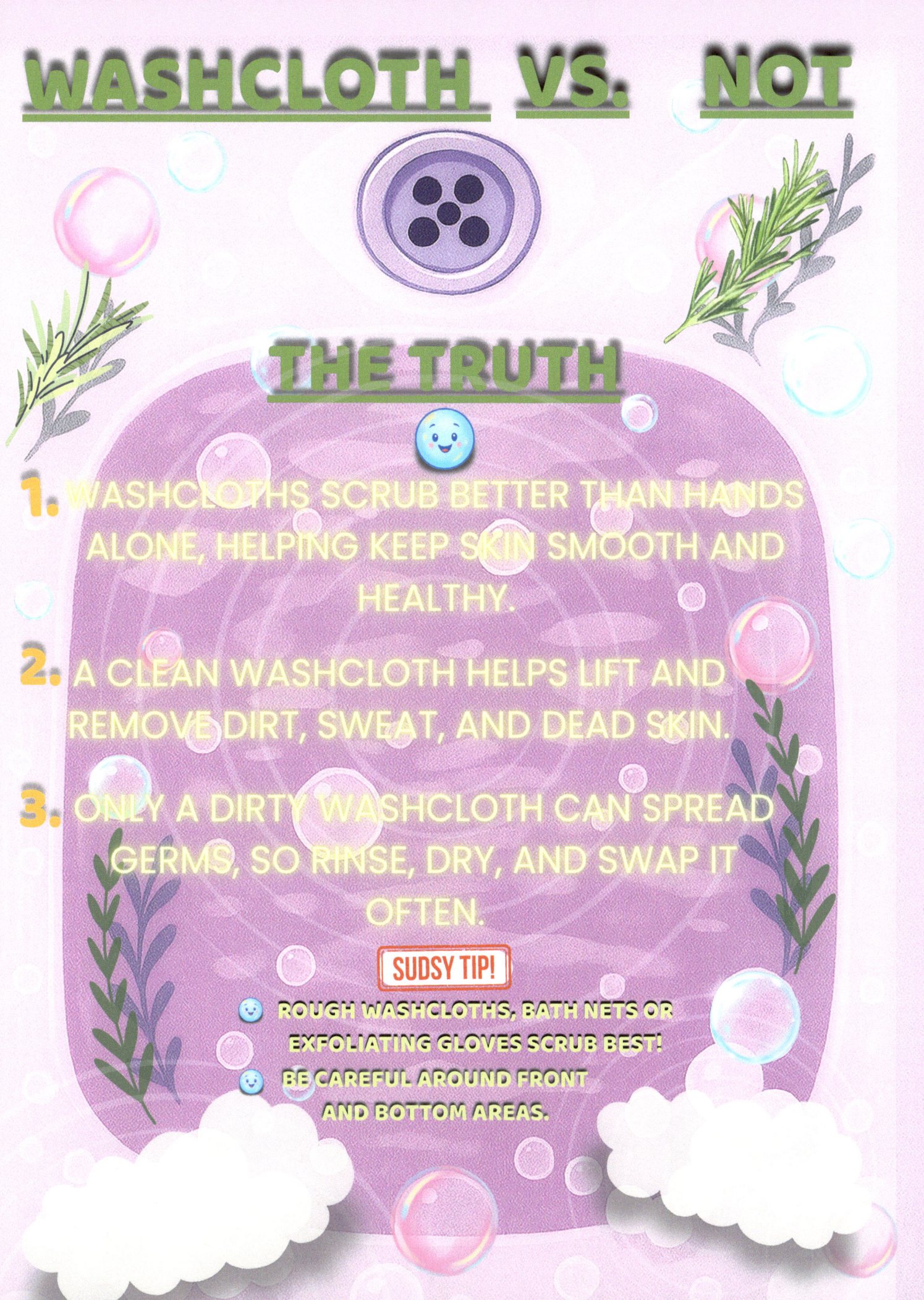

AREAS AND STEPS WE FORGET

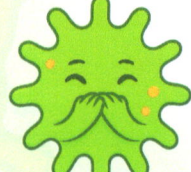 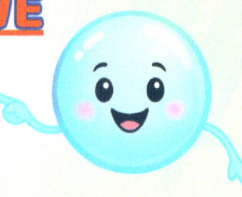

MOUTH
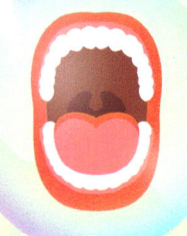

NOSE
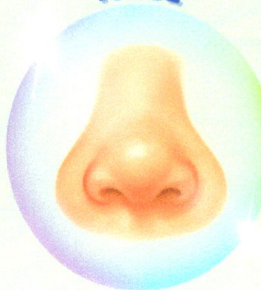

EARS
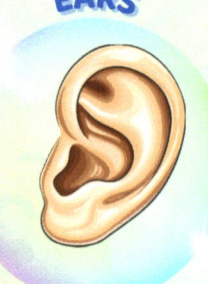

- FLOSS.
- BRUSH BEHIND THE TEETH AND GUM LINE.
- RINSE VERY WELL.
- GARGLE.
- USE MOUTHWASH OR MOUTHRINSE.

- BLOW NOSE AND CLEAN EACH NOSTRIL AFTER BRUSHING AND RINSING.
- BLOW NOSE AND CLEAN NOSTRILS THROUOUT THE DAY.

- WASH THE ENTIRE EAR, FRONT AND BACK.
- CLEAN OUT WAX DAILY.

SUDSY TIP!

EVEN IF YOU WASH YOUR EARS IN THE BATH OR SHOWER, DON'T FORGET THE BACK OF THEM DURING THE DAY, ESPECIALLY IF IT'S HOT OR YOU'VE BEEN SWEATING. GERMIES LOVE TO HANG OUT THERE AND WILL MAKE IT *VERY* STINKY! A GENTLE WIPE WITH ALCOHOL AND A LITTLE COCONUT OIL AFTER HELPS KEEP THINGS FRESH AND CLEAN.

FINGERNAILS
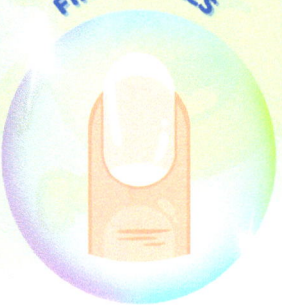

EYES
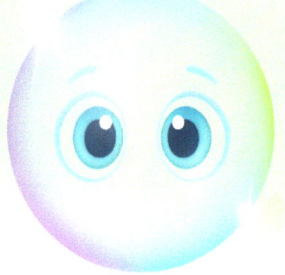

BOTTOM
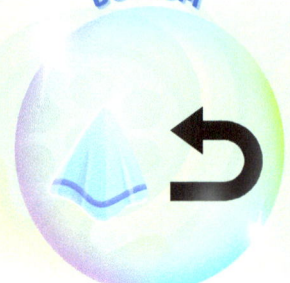

- SCRUB UNDER YOUR NAILS.
- CLEAR AWAY DIRT AND GRIME WITH SOAP, WATER AND A NAIL BRUSH.

- CHECK EYES WHEN WASHING FACE.
- MAKE SURE SLEEP AND CRUST IS WASHED AWAY.
- CHECK THROUGHOUT THE DAY.

- WIPE YOUR BOTTOM UNTIL THE TOILET PAPER OR WIPES STAY CLEAN AND WHITE, EVEN BEFORE A BATH OR SHOWER.
- WIPE FRONT TO BACK.

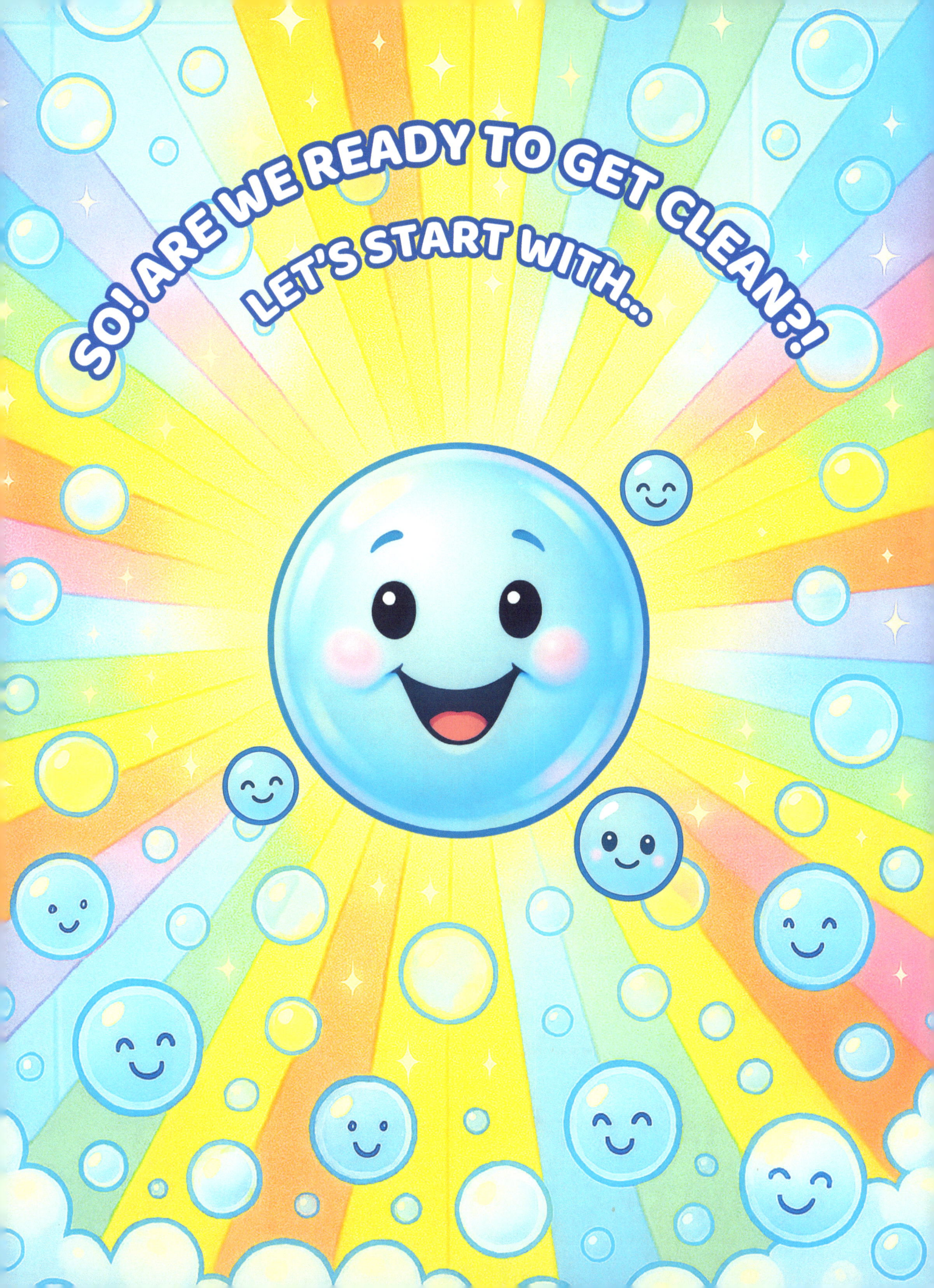

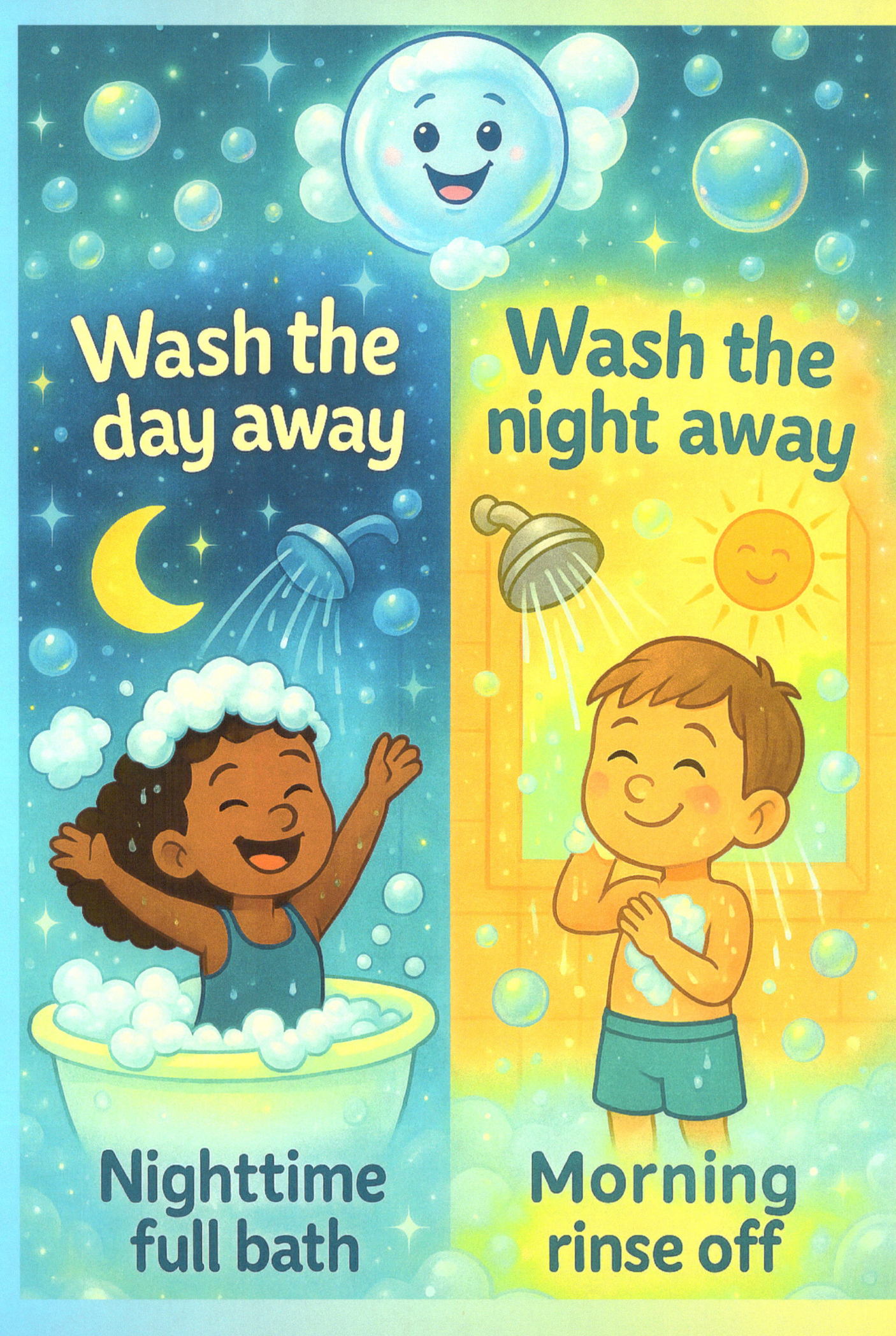

Q&A: Why Bathe Twice a Day?

Q Why Bathe Twice a Day?

A Bathing at night helps wash away the day's dirt and Germies while a quick rinse in the morning freshens you up and gets you ready to shine!

Q What's the science behind soap anyway?

A Soap molecules grab onto dirt, oil, and Germies when they come into contact with water. One end of the soap sticks to grime, while the other sticks to the water, kind of like a two sided magnet. That's how soap lifts all the Germies off your skin so water can wash them all away!

Q Can't I just use wipes, sprays, oils, or creams instead of bathing?

A Nope! Wipes, sprays, oils, and creams don't remove dirt, sweat, or Germies like soap and water can. They're only meant for emergencies or quick fresh ups only. These quick fixes might cover up smells but for some, they may cause burning, itching, or even infections. Oils and creams can even trap dirt under a greasy layer, making it harder for our skin to breathe. You might smell nice for a minute, but underneath? you are still dirty. Scrub your skin every day to keep it clean and healthy.

Q But I don't stink so why do I still need to wash every day?

A Your body sheds dead skin, makes sweat, and collects germs every single day even if you don't smell it yet. A clean or neutral smelling body can still be carrying bacteria that causes rashes, acne, and odor later. Prevention is everything.

Q What if I don't feel like it or don't have time?

A You don't have to take a long bath or shower, but you do need to wash your key areas daily: face, neck, behind the ears, underarms, your bottom, including your front and creases, LEGS, feet and between toes. A quick wash with soap and water using a washcloth, exfoliating gloves or net, works great! Clean habits = healthy body!

Q What about people who say soap is bad for your skin?

A Some soaps can be too harsh, especially scented or drying ones. But there are gentle, moisturizing soaps made for daily use. The key is to wash with clean water and a cleanser that lifts away dirt. No soap = no real clean.

So, in short, bathing twice a day helps your skin stay healthy, your body smell fresh, and your whole self feel squeaky clean. And when you feel clean, you shine from the inside out!

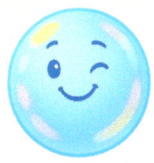

WASH the DAY AWAY

WASH the NIGHT AWAY

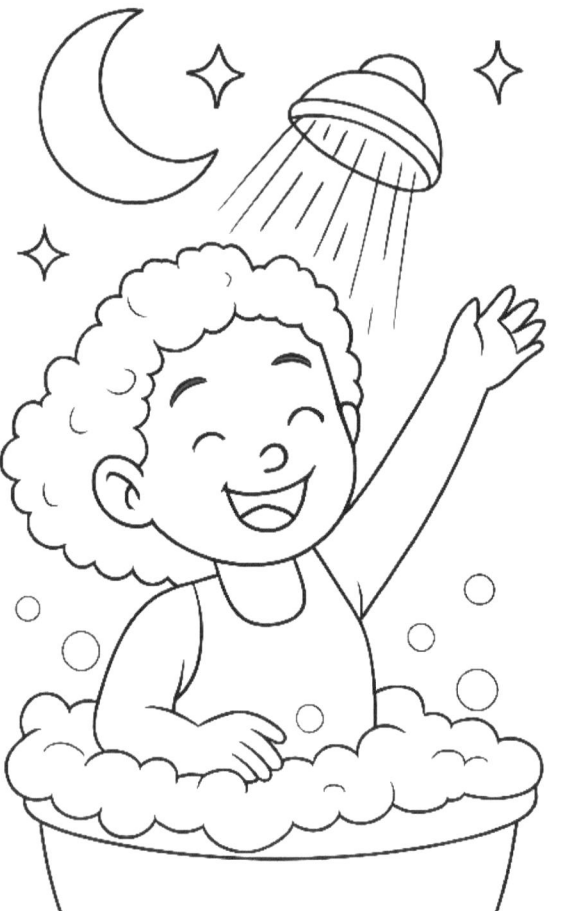

Nighttime full bath

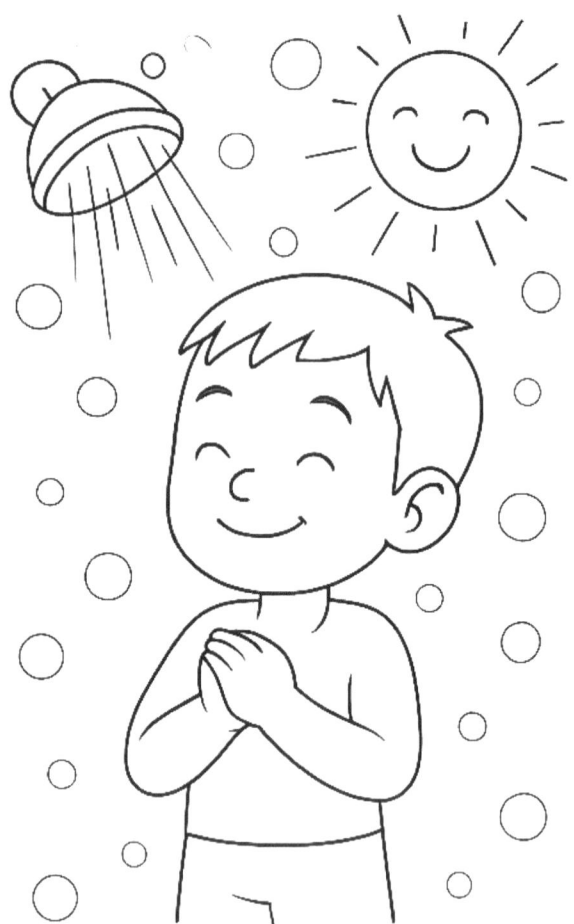

Morning rinse off

WHERE and HOW to Wash!

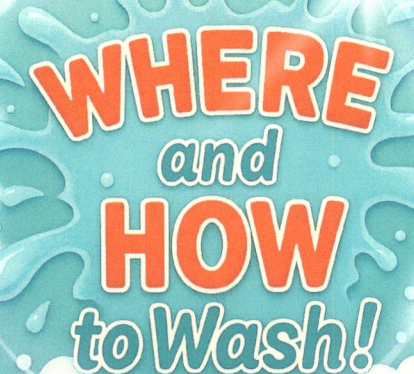

TOOLS YOU MAY NEED:

 SHAMPOO AND CONDITIONER.

 SOAP OR BODYWASH.

 WASHCLOTH OR EXFOLIATING GLOVES.

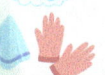 LARGE BATH TOWEL/BATH ROBE.

BEFORE YOU BEGIN:

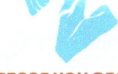 WIPE YOUR BOTTOM FROM FRONT TO BACK BEFORE GETTING IN THE BATH OR SHOWER. ✓

 USE FRESH TOILET PAPER OR A WIPE EACH TIME. KEEP WIPING UNTIL IT STAYS WHITE AND CLEAN. ✓

 THIS HELPS KEEP YUCKY STUFF AND GERMIES FROM GETTING STUCK IN YOUR TOWEL OR ON YOUR BODY WHEN YOU BATHE OR SHOWER. ✓

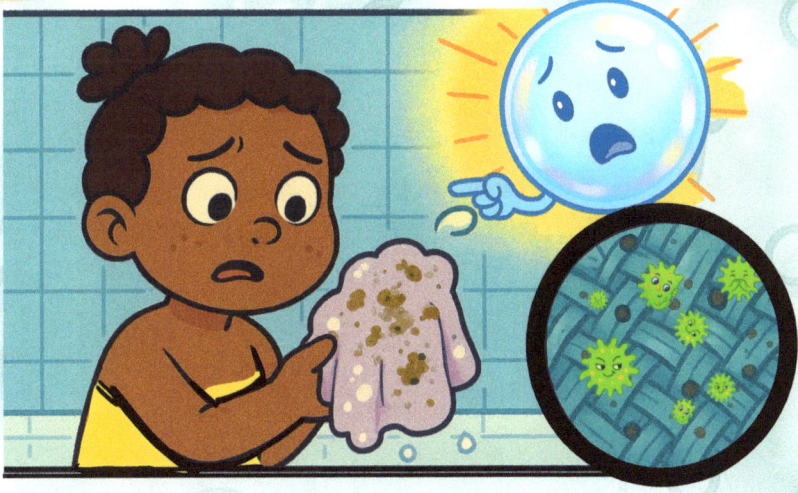

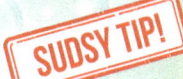 **SUDSY TIP!**

HAIR SUDS AREN'T BODYWASH! SUDS FROM WASHING YOUR HAIR DO NOT CLEAN YOUR BODY. DIRT AND DEAD SKIN CELLS HAVE TO BE SCRUBBED AWAY!

THIS IS WHAT CAN HAPPEN WHEN WE DON'T WIPE BEFORE BATHTIME! EVEN IF WE RINSE THIS TOWEL OUT WITH BODY SOAP AND WATER, THERE WILL STILL BE YUCKIES AND GERMIES STUCK IN OUR TOWEL! DO YOU WANT THIS ON YOUR BODY?

Step 1: Hair

- If showering, use shampoo.
- Rub your scalp gently.
- Smooth hair down.
- Rinse downward.

Step 2: Face

- Use clean hands or a clean washcloth.
- Wash your face with mild soap or face wash.
- Gently clean around your eyes, nose, and mouth.
- Rinse well.

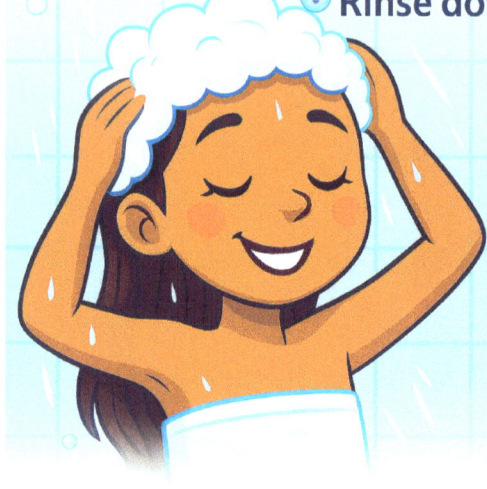

Step 3: Upper Body

- Rinse your towel, add fresh soap.
- Wash in and behind your ears.
- Scrub your neck, arms, chest, and belly.
- Don't forget your belly button.

Step 4: Back

- Rinse your towel add fresh soap.
- Scrub your back as best you can.
- Ask for help if you need it.

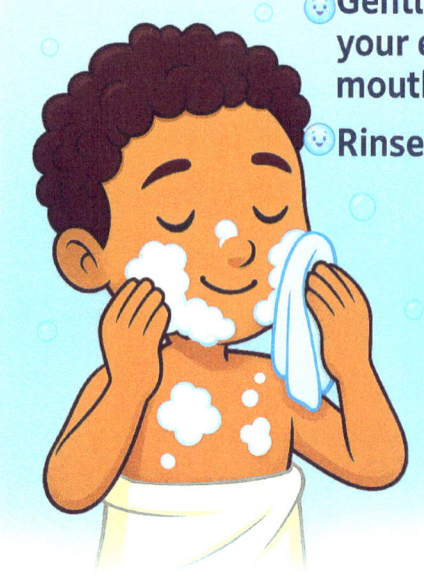
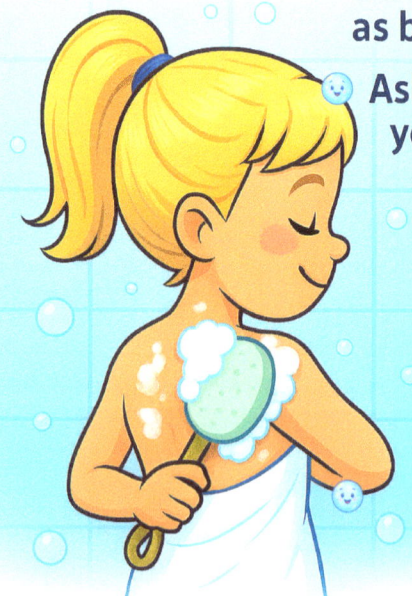

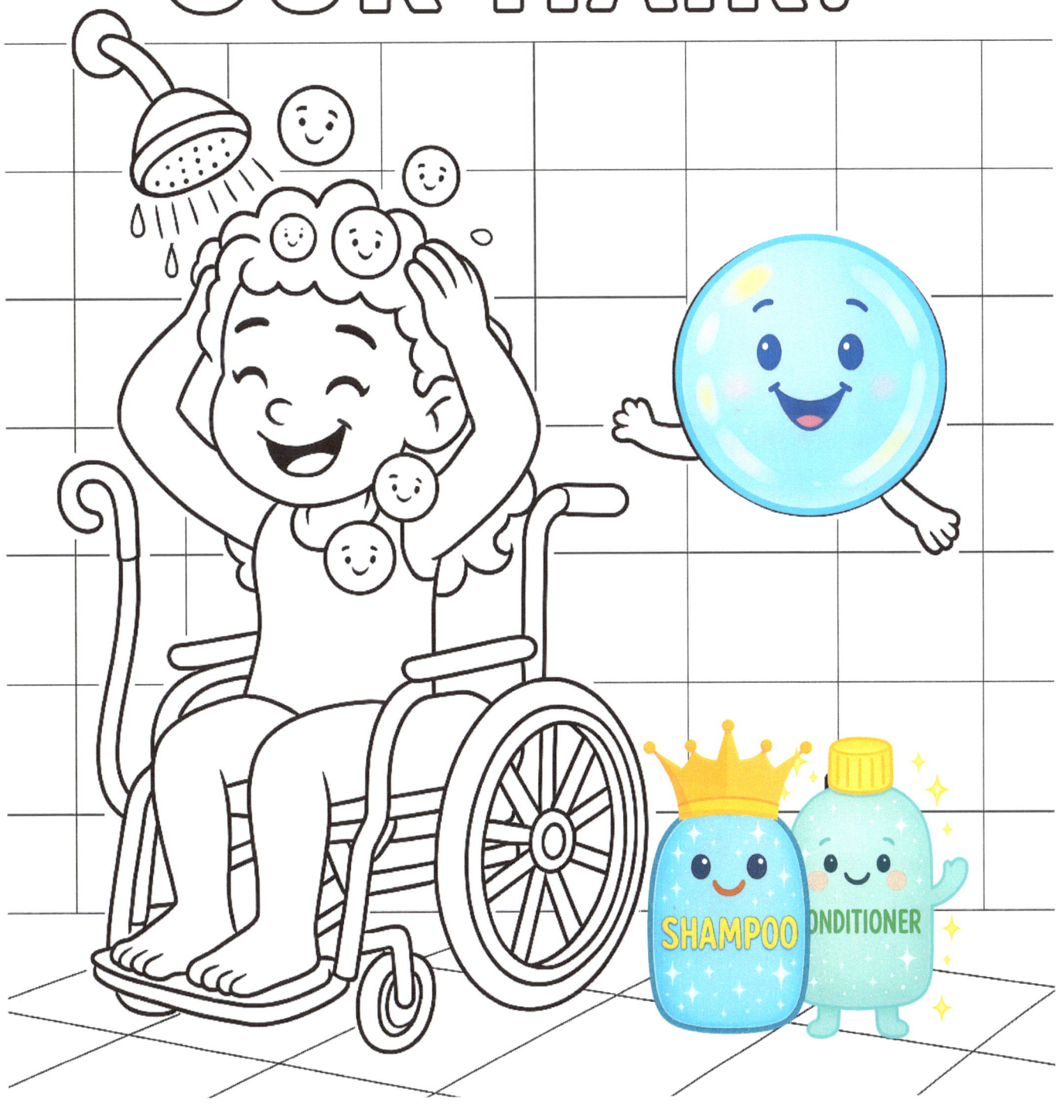

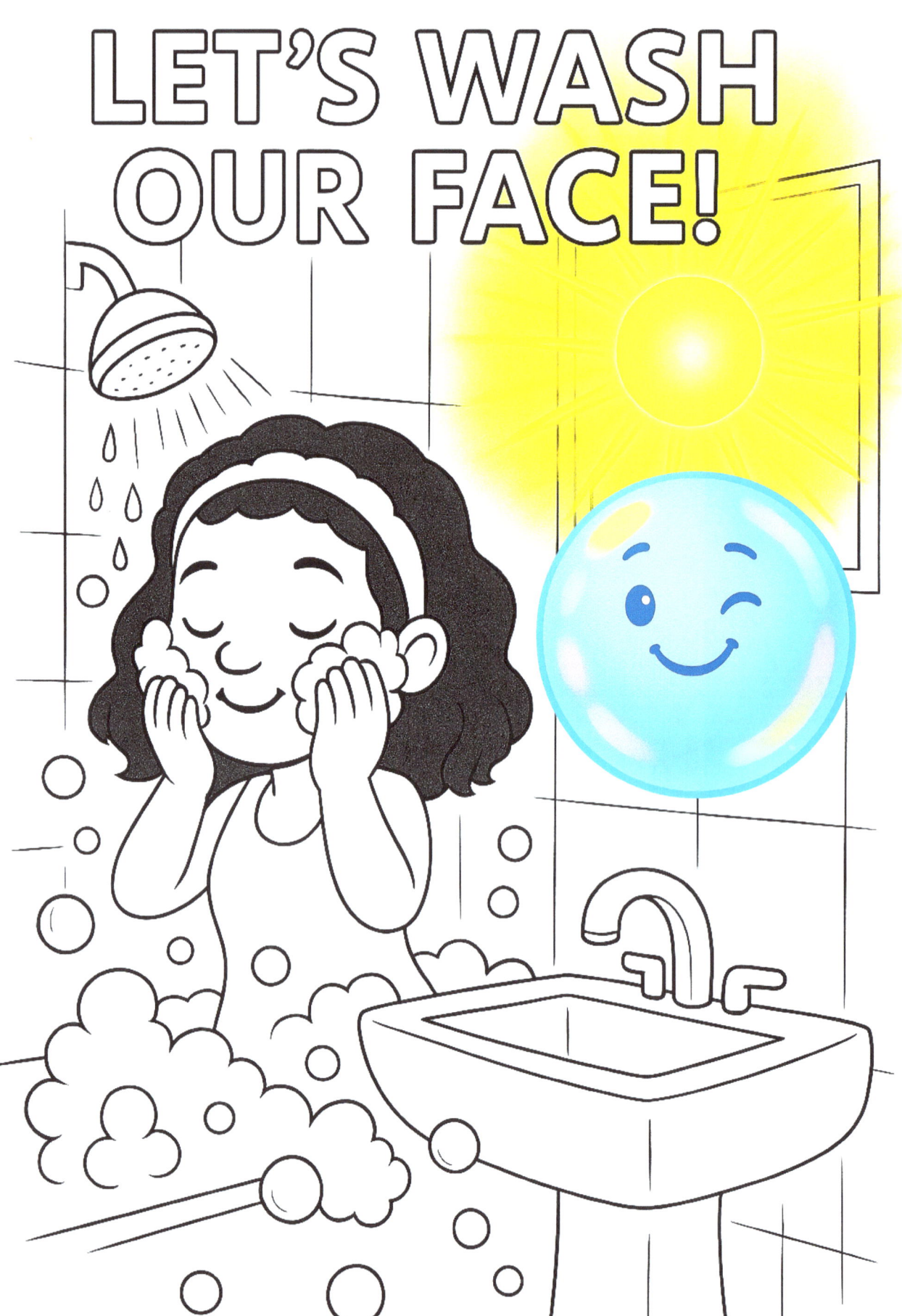

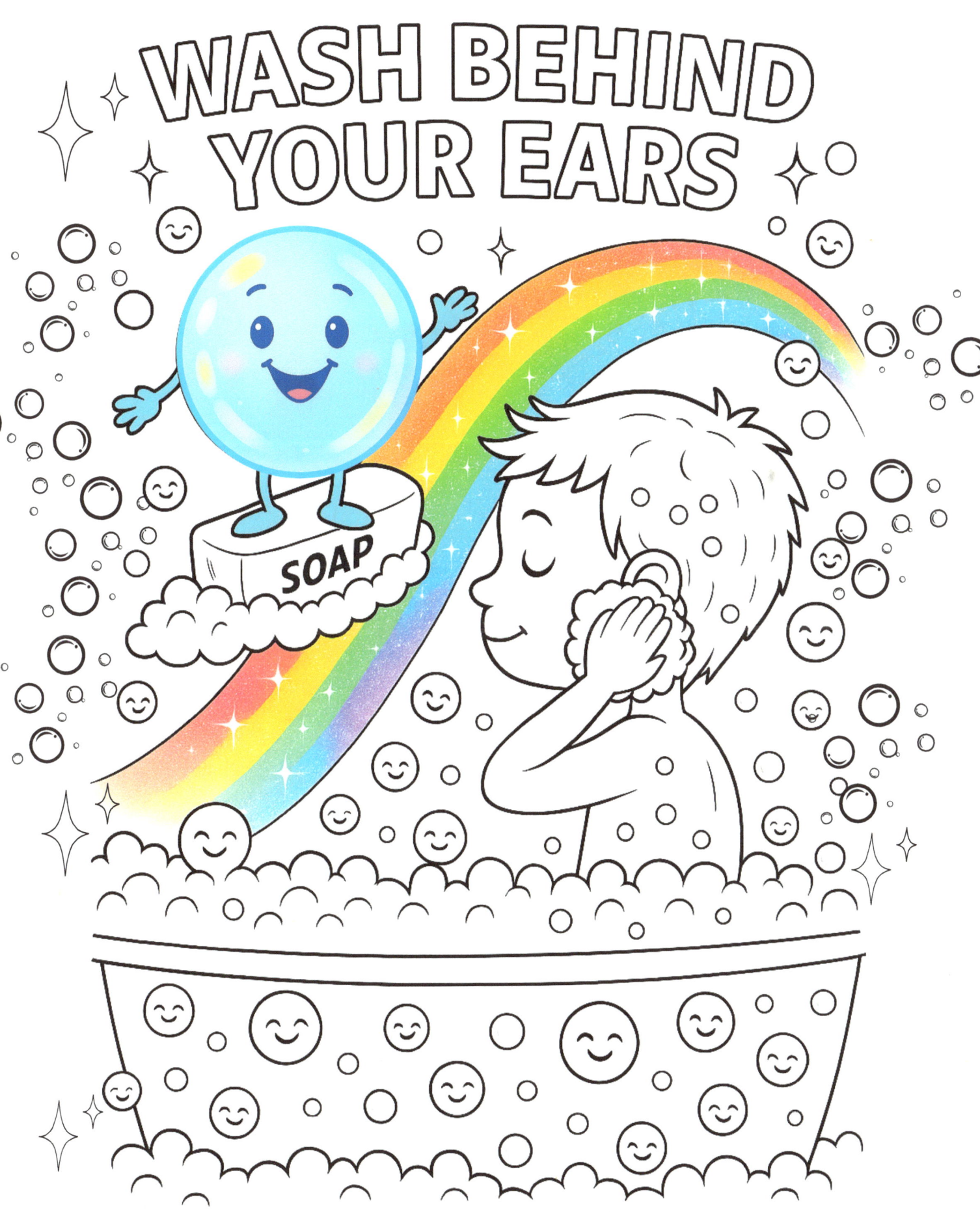

LET'S WASH OUR NECK!

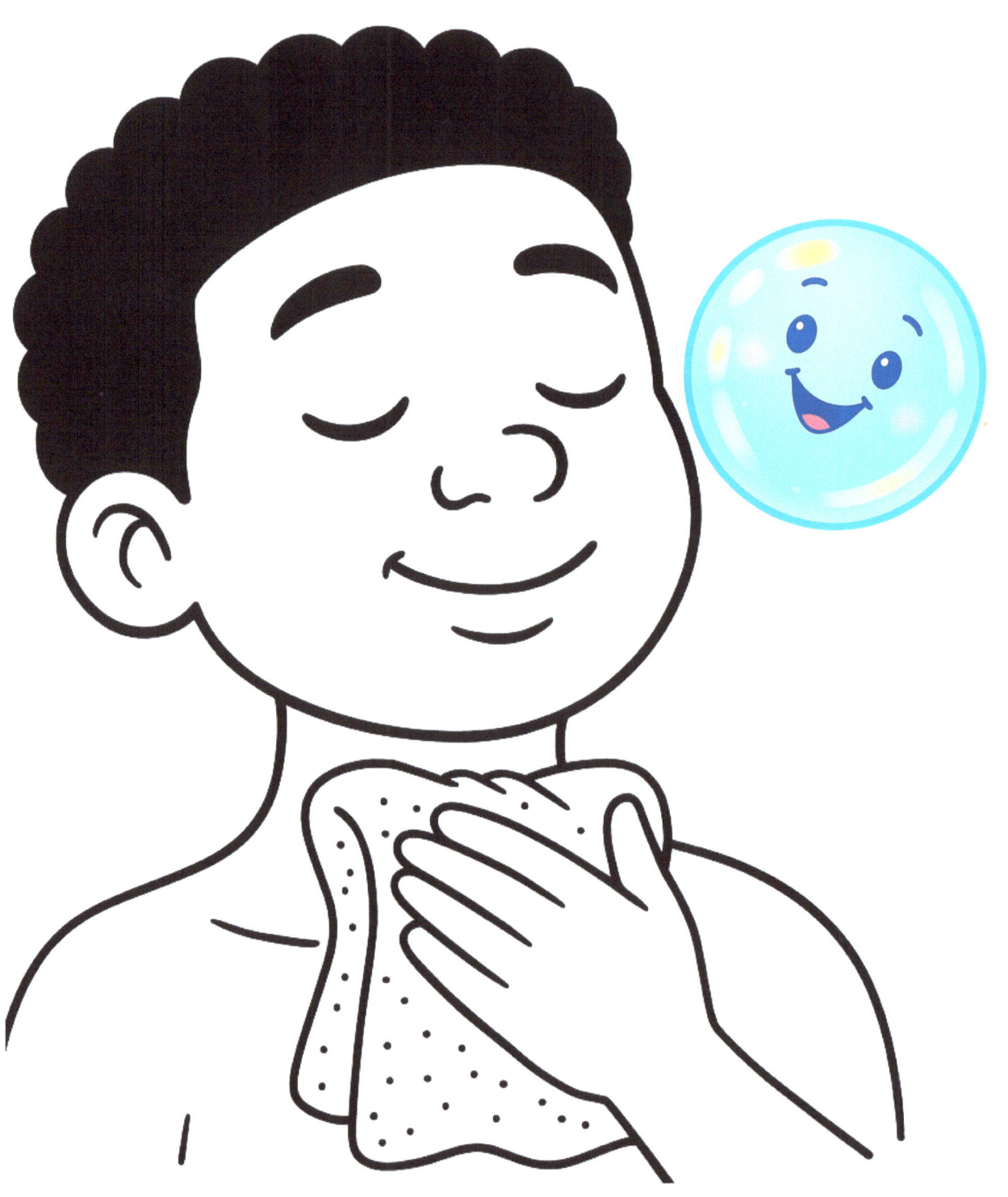

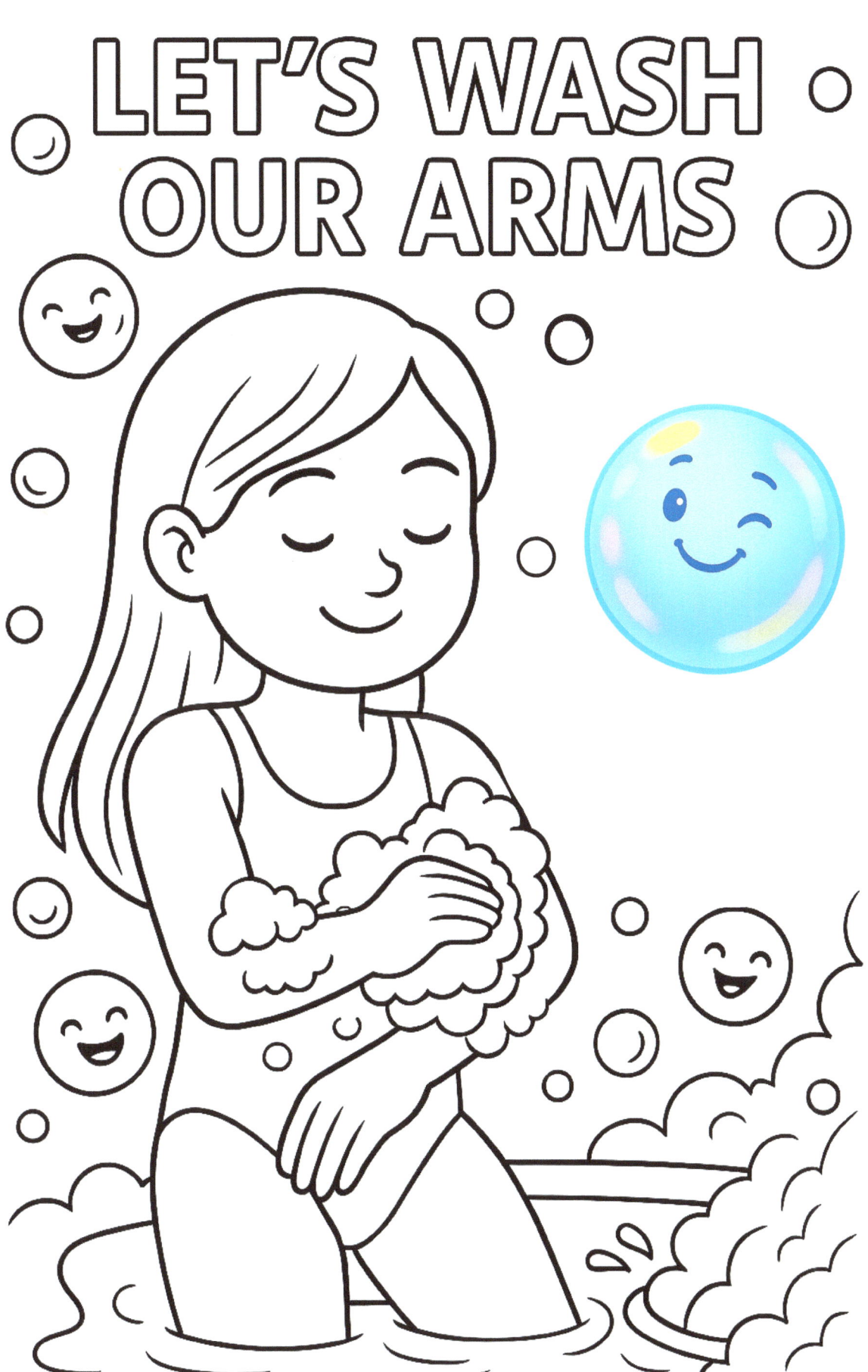

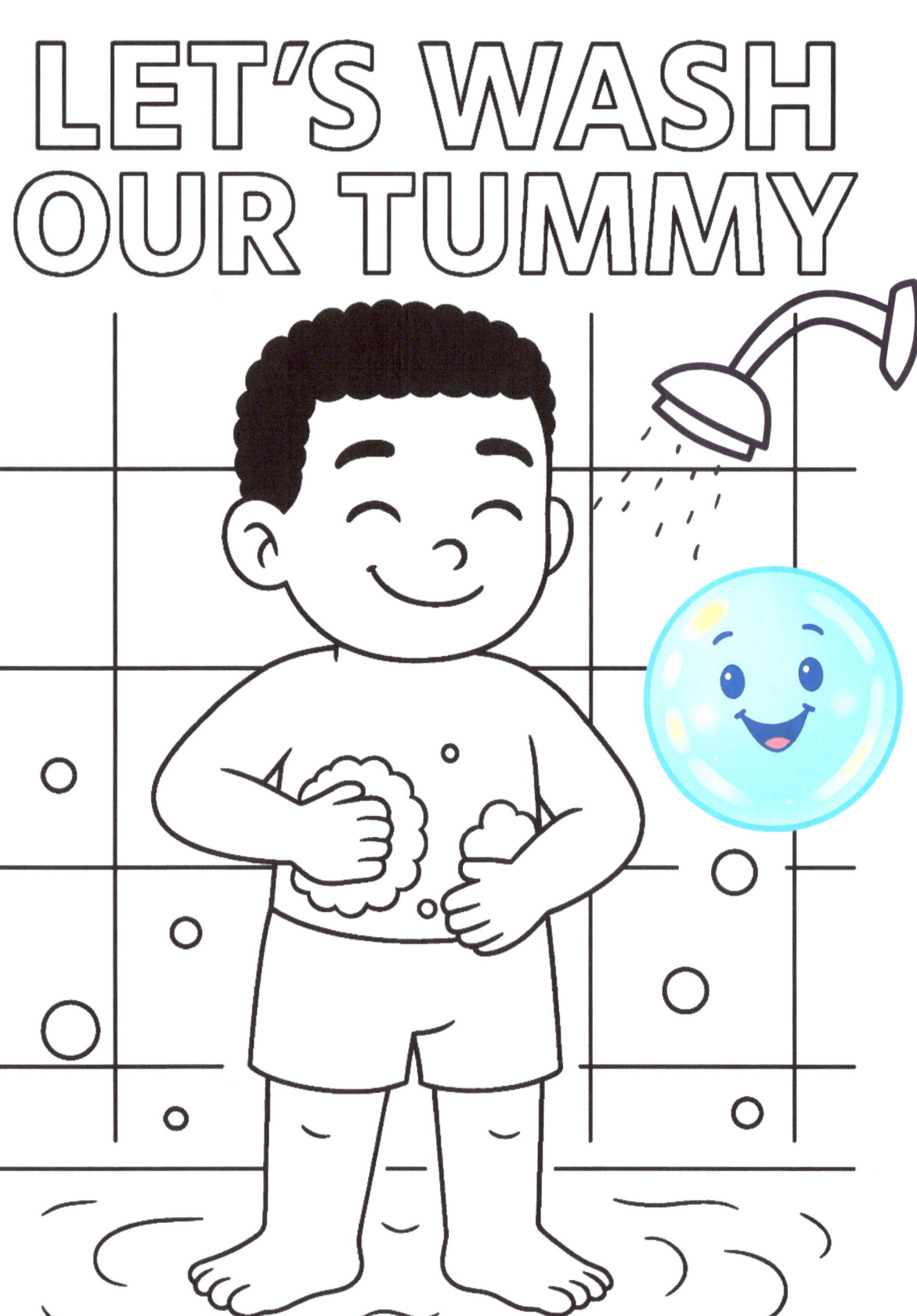

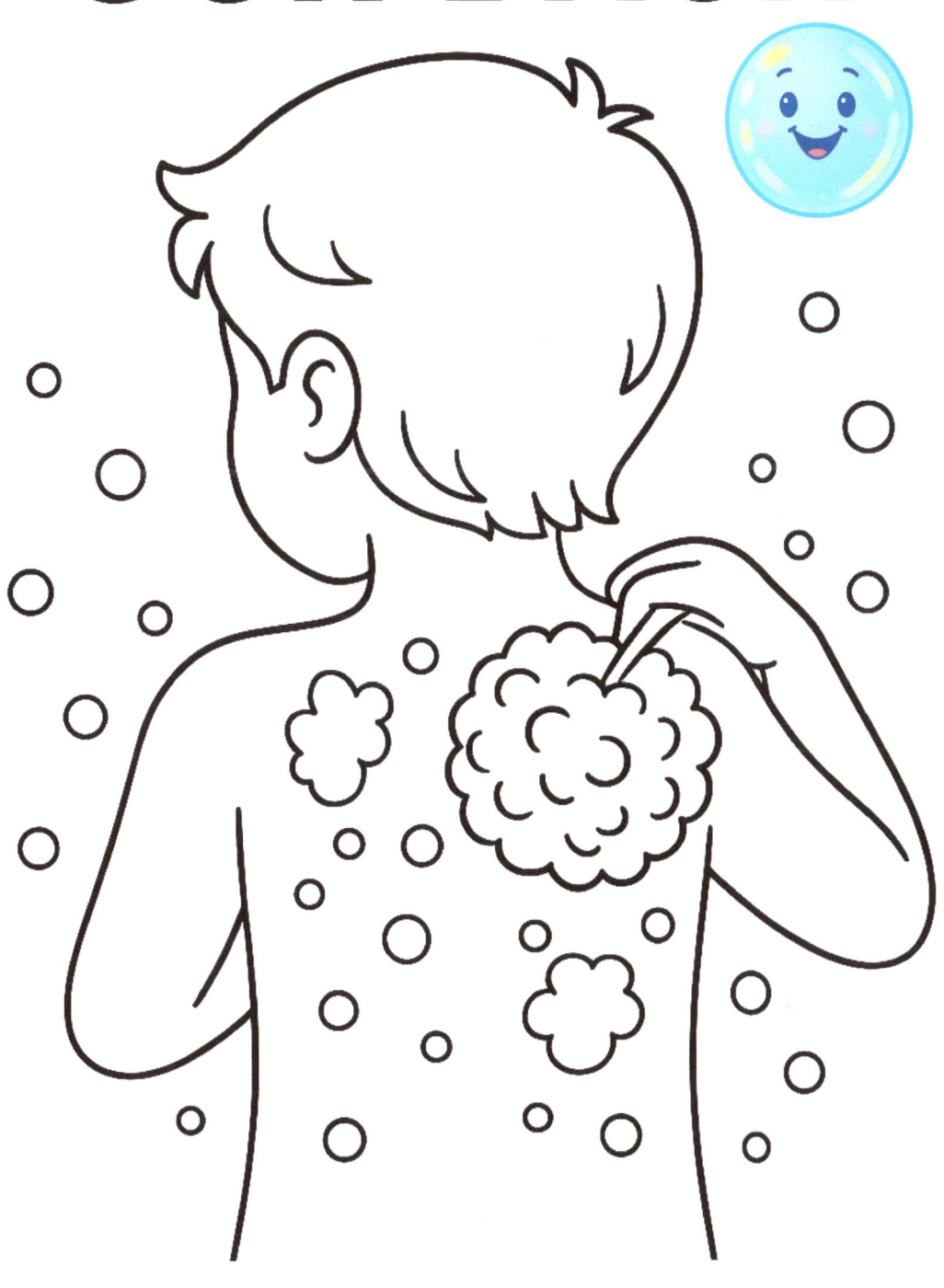

Step 5: Underarms

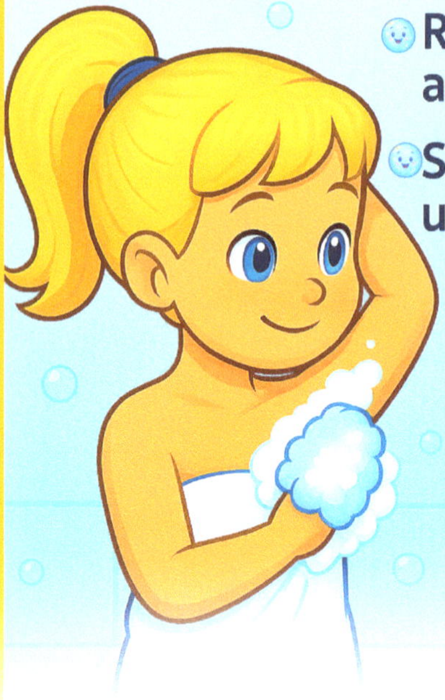

- Rinse your towel add fresh soap.
- Scrub your underarms.
- Scrub under both arms very well.

Step 6: Legs

- Rinse your towel add fresh soap.
- Scrub your legs on all sides, front, back, and sides.
- Don't forget your ankles. Scrub very well.

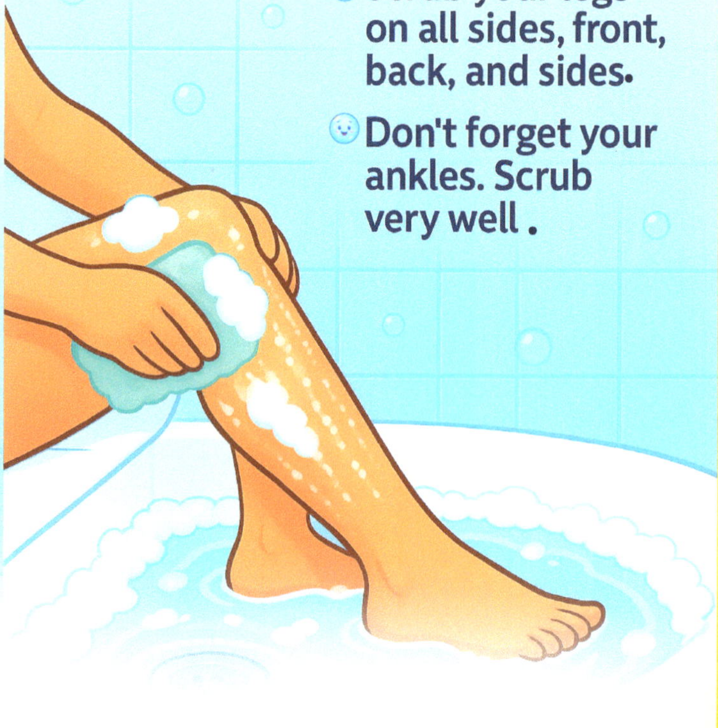

STEP 7 **IS EXTRA SPECIAL!**

IT'S TIME TO LEARN HOW TO PROPERLY WASH OUR BOTTOM.
AND GUESS WHAT?! WE'VE GOT A VERY HELPFUL FRIEND TO GUIDE US!

COME ON! FOLLOW US TO BEGIN!

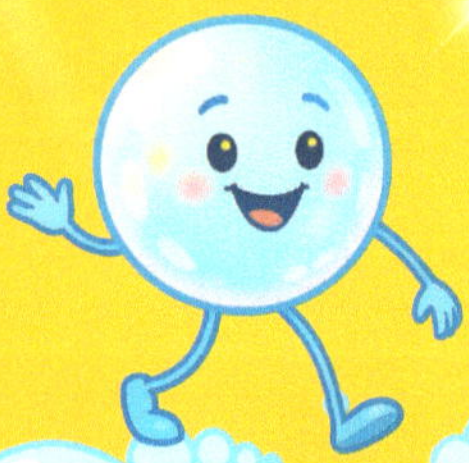

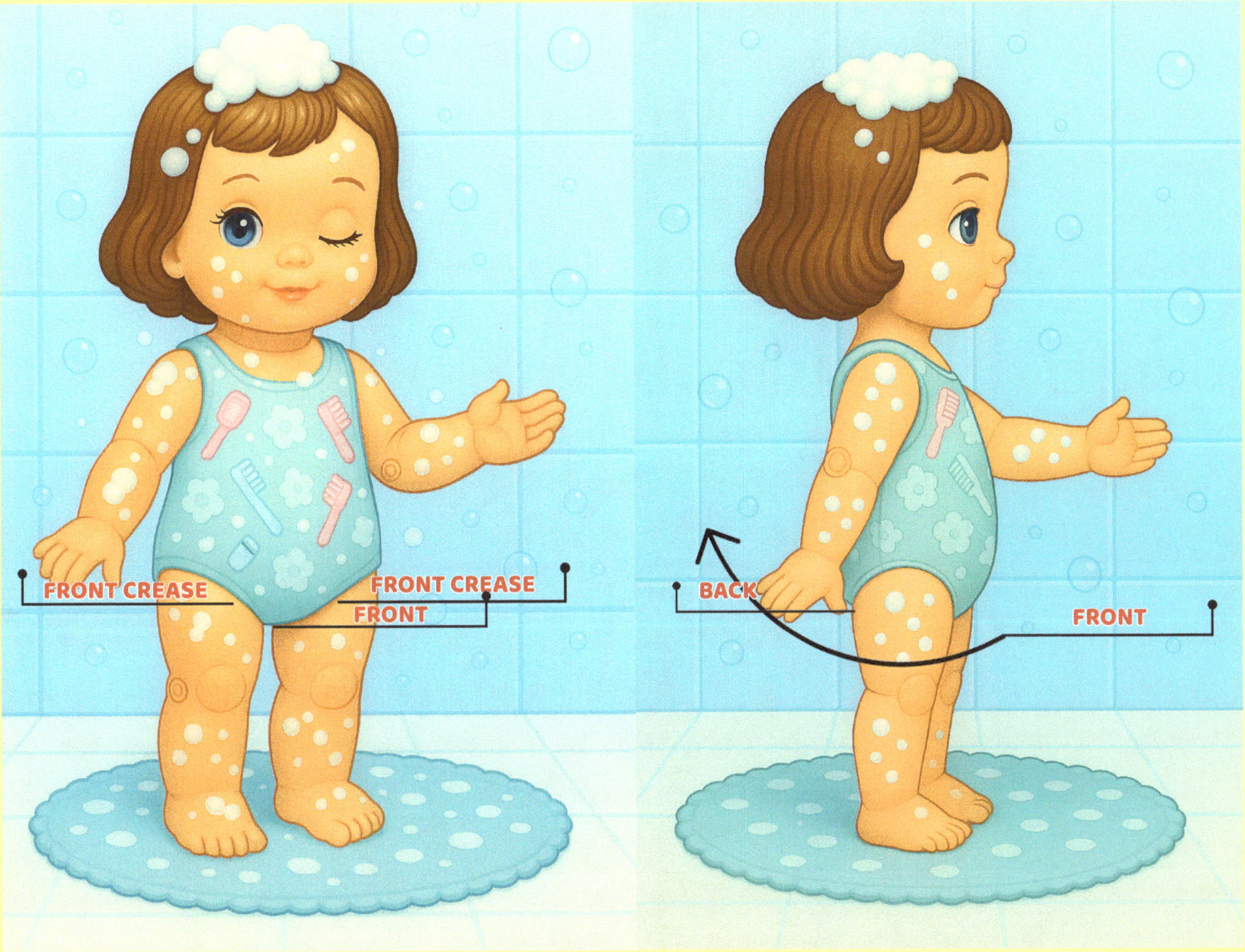

It's practice time! Let's learn with our helper doll!

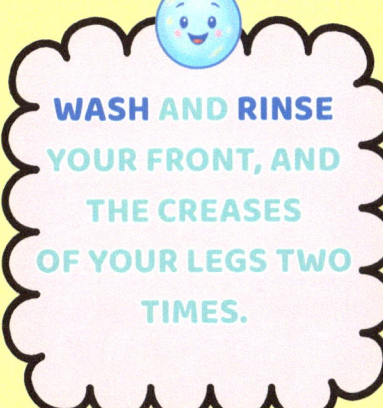

WASH AND RINSE YOUR FRONT, AND THE CREASES OF YOUR LEGS TWO TIMES.

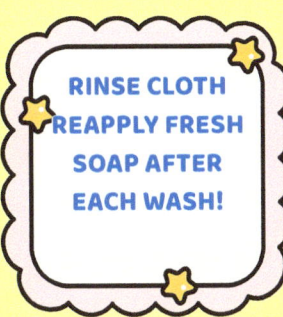

RINSE CLOTH REAPPLY FRESH SOAP AFTER EACH WASH!

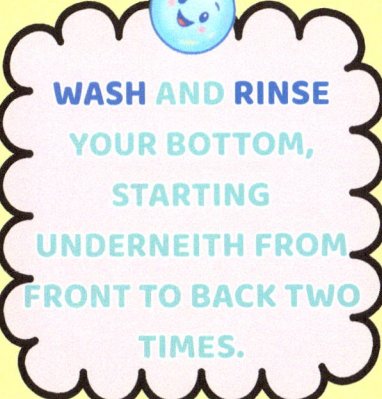

WASH AND RINSE YOUR BOTTOM, STARTING UNDERNEITH FROM FRONT TO BACK TWO TIMES.

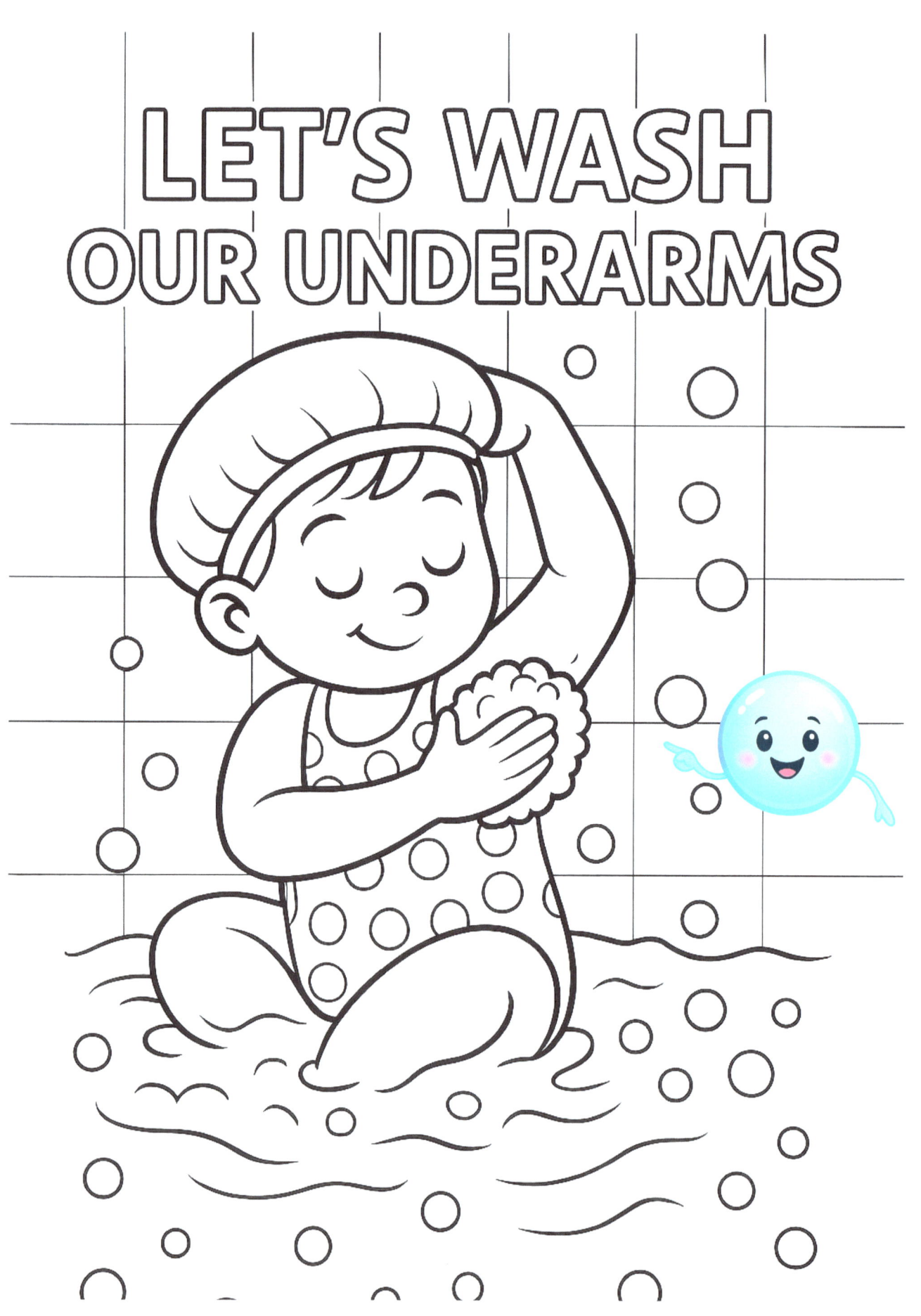

LET'S WASH OUR LEGS

STEP 8
FEET

- RINSE YOUR TOWEL, ADD FRESH SOAP.
- WASH YOUR FEET, TOP BOTTON AND SIDES.
- SCRUB BETWEEN EVERY TOE.

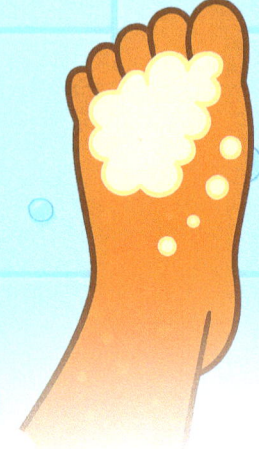
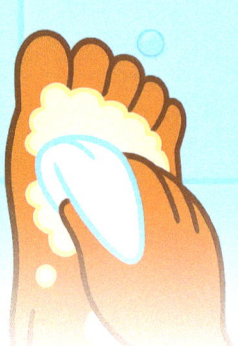

STEP 9
FINGERNAILS

- CLEAN UNDER YOUR NAILS.
- USE A NAIL SCRUBBER OR SCRAPER.

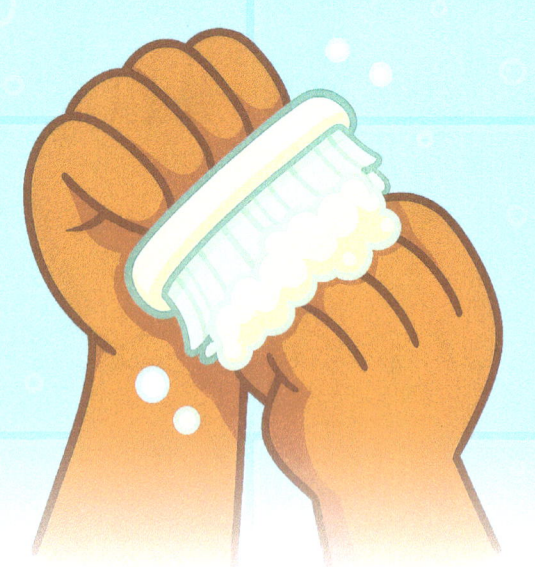

STEP 10
FINAL RINSE

- RINSE OFF ONE LAST TIME.
- MAKE SURE NO SOAP IS LEFT BEHIND.

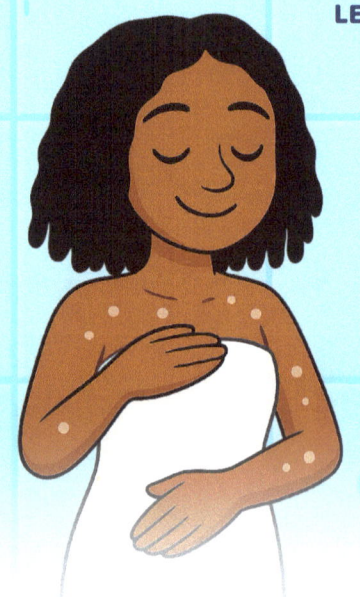

STEP 11
TEETH

- FLOSS YOUR TEETH.
- BRUSH YOUR TEETH ON ALL SIDES: FRONT, SIDES, TOP AND BOTTOM, BRUSH BEHIND YOUR TEETH AND SCRUB YOUR TONGUE TOO!

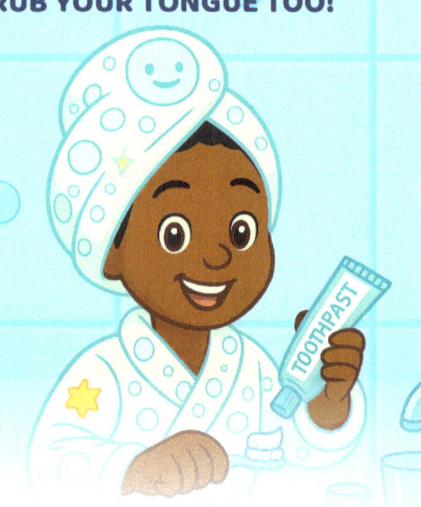

ALL DONE! YOU DID A GREAT JOB!

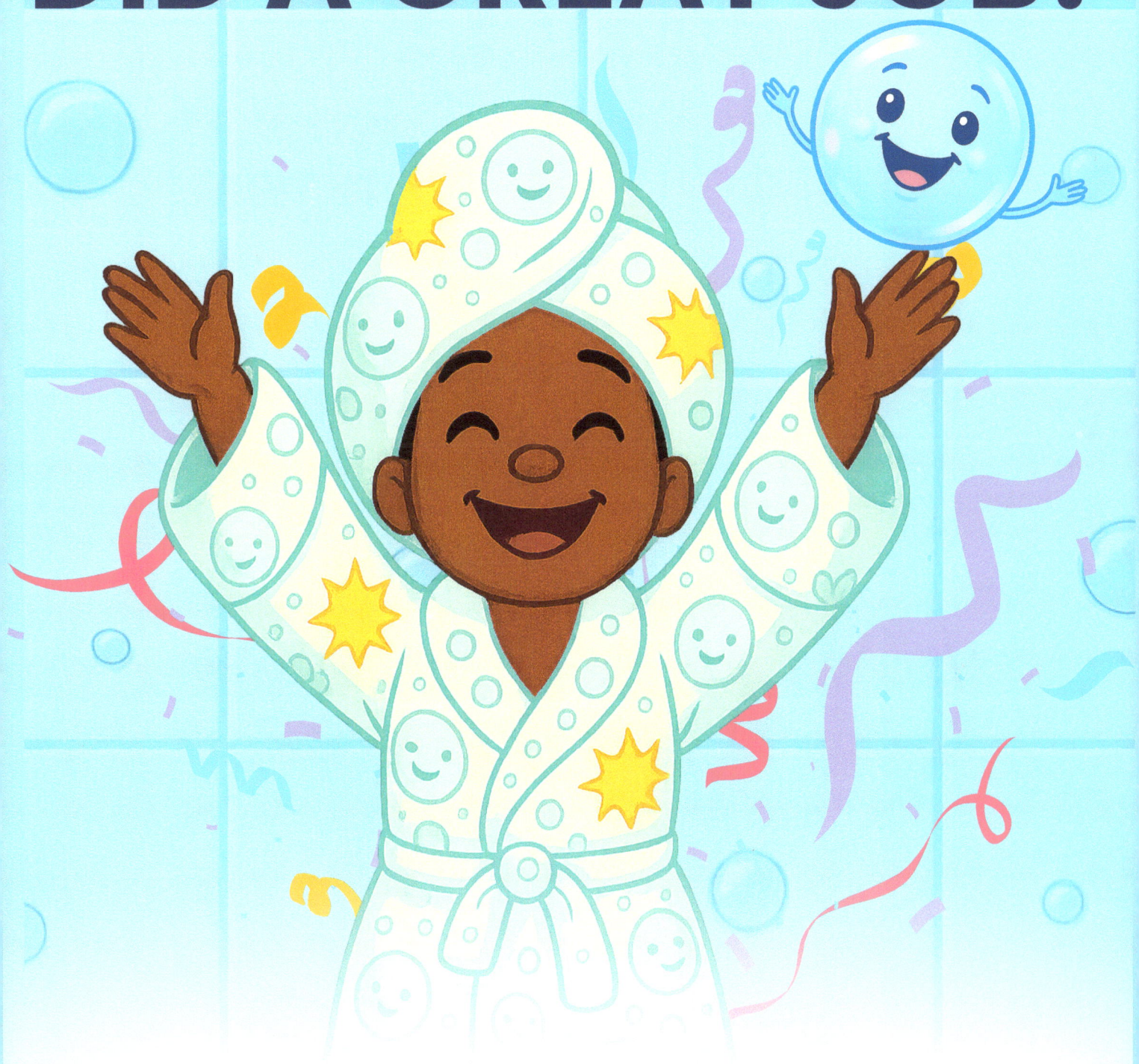

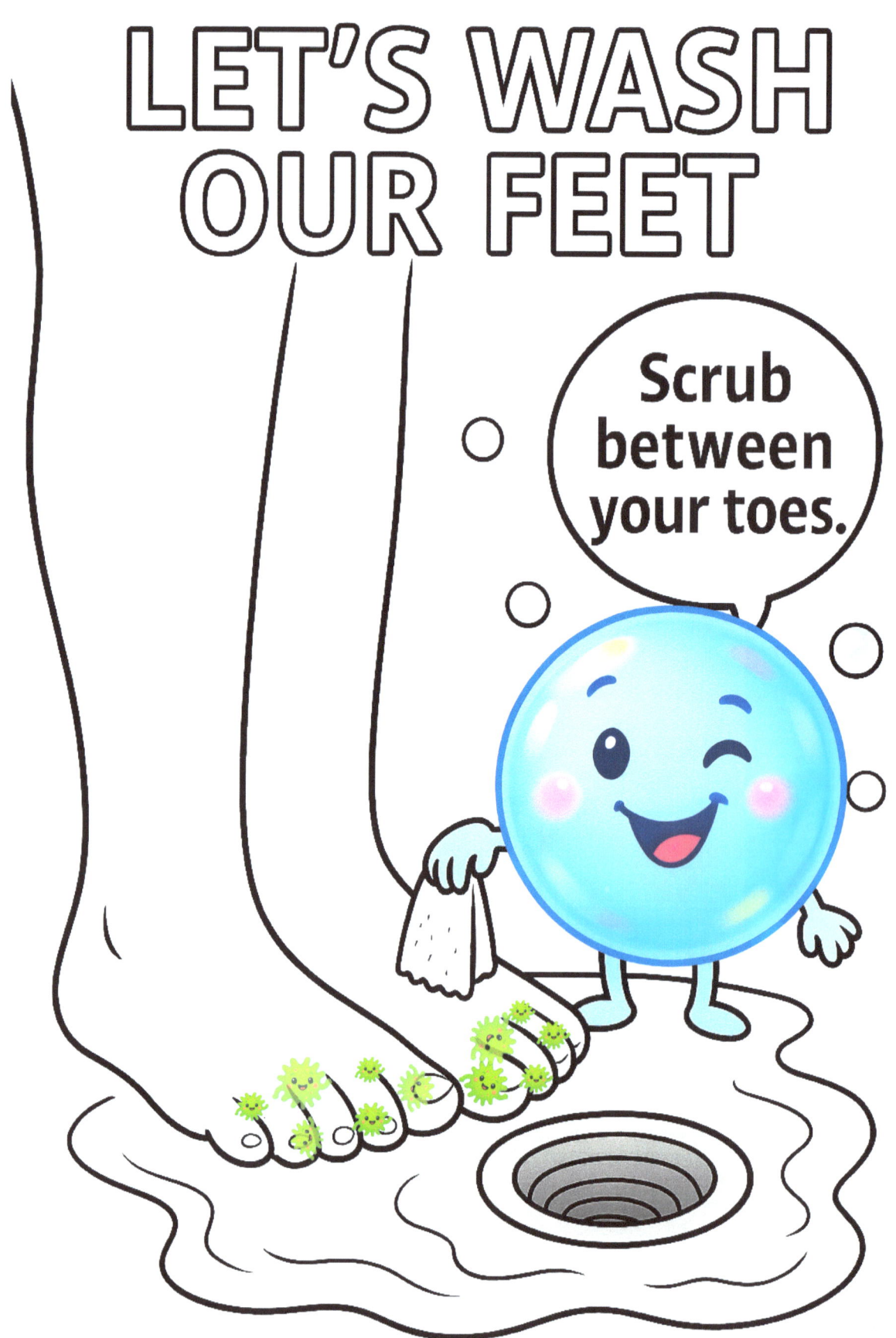

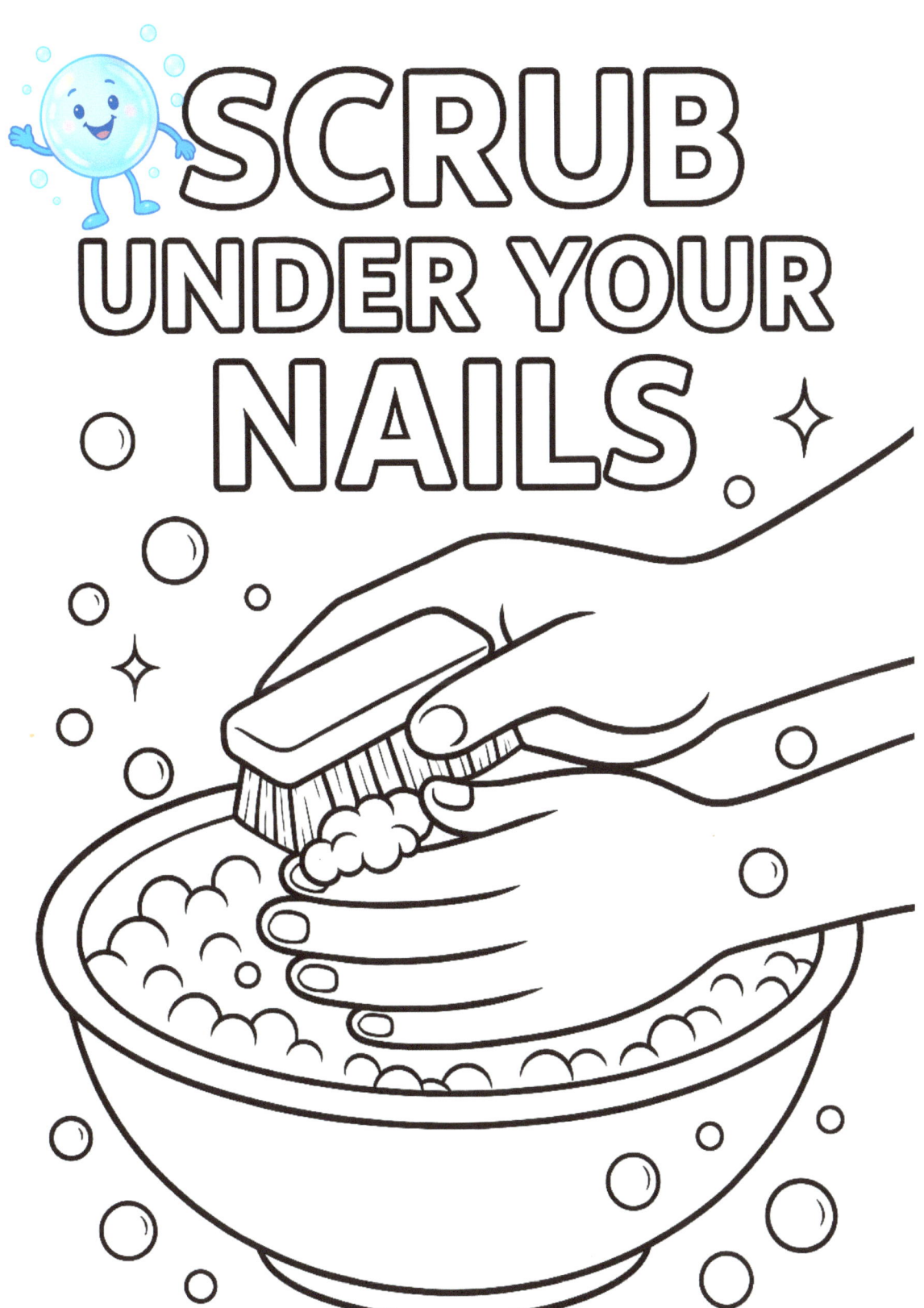

FLOSS YOUR TEETH!

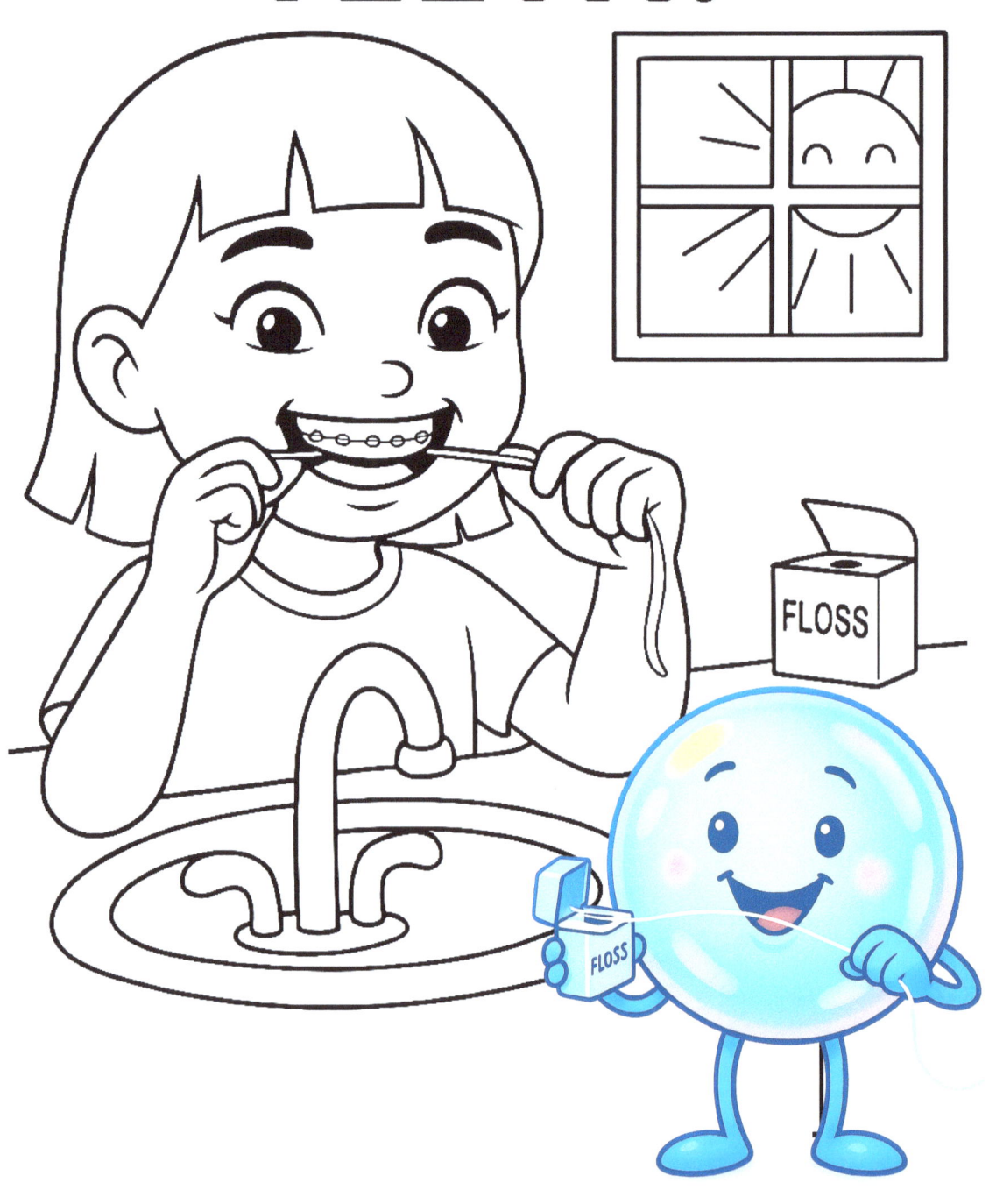

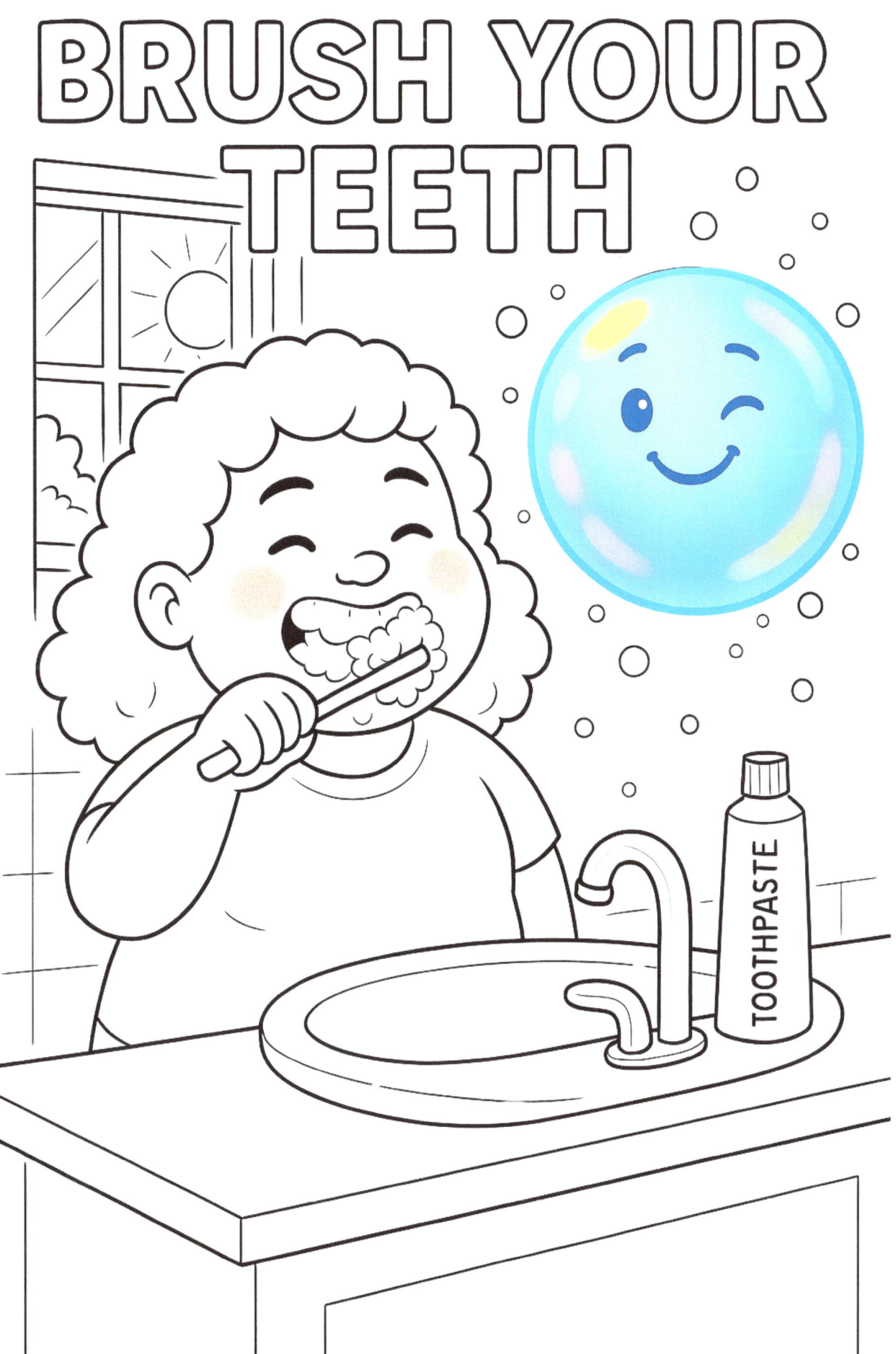

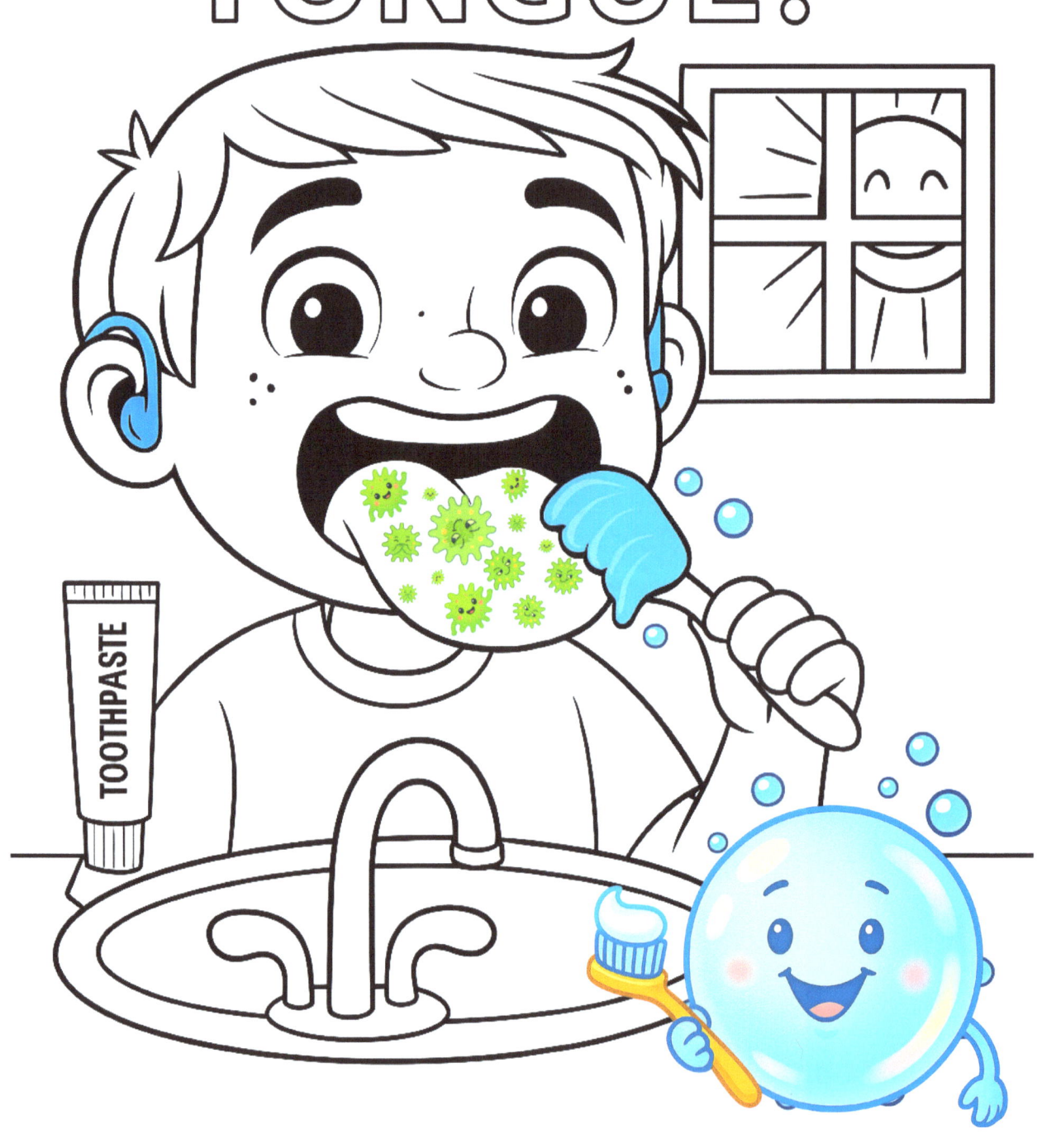

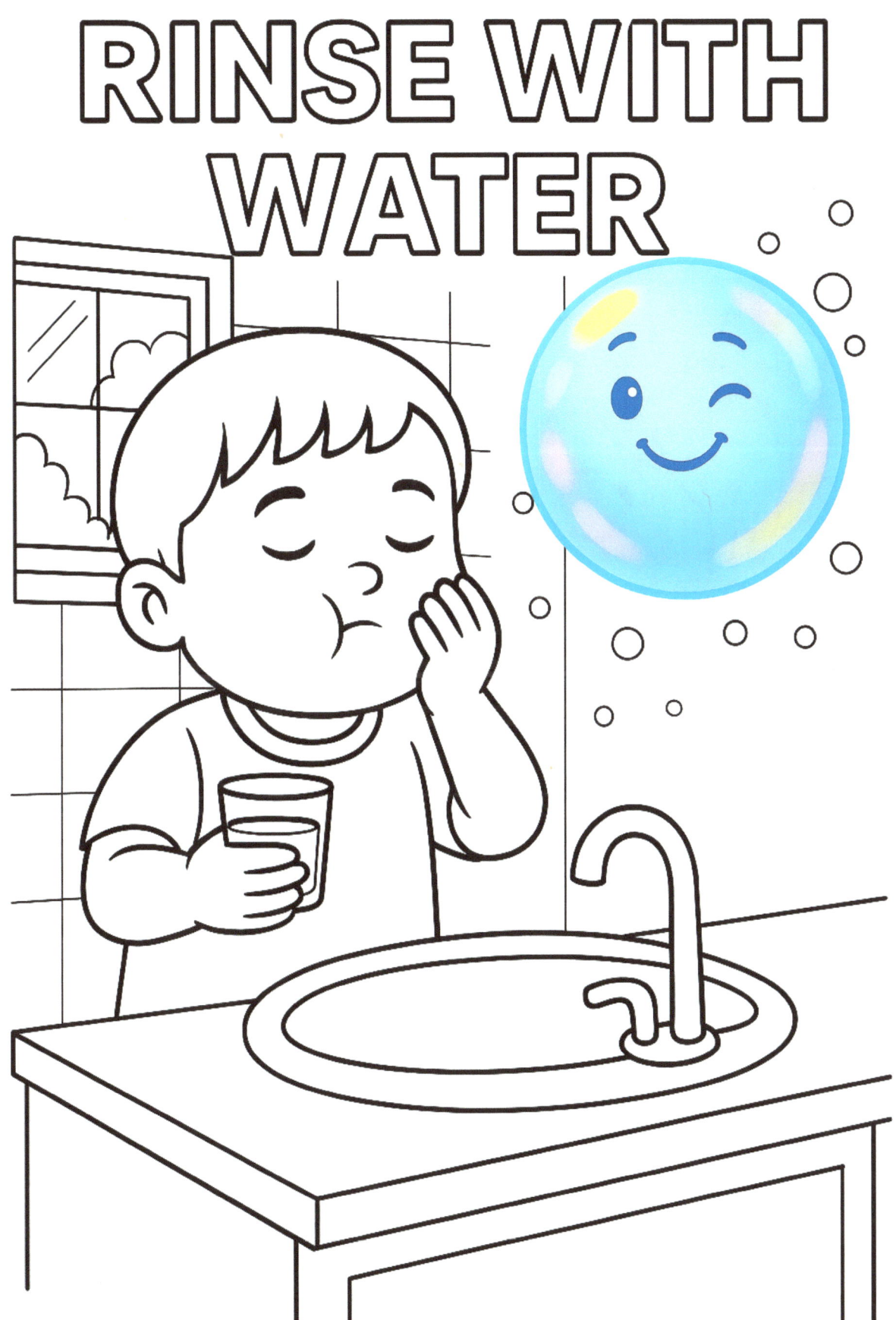

RINSE WITH MOUTHWASH

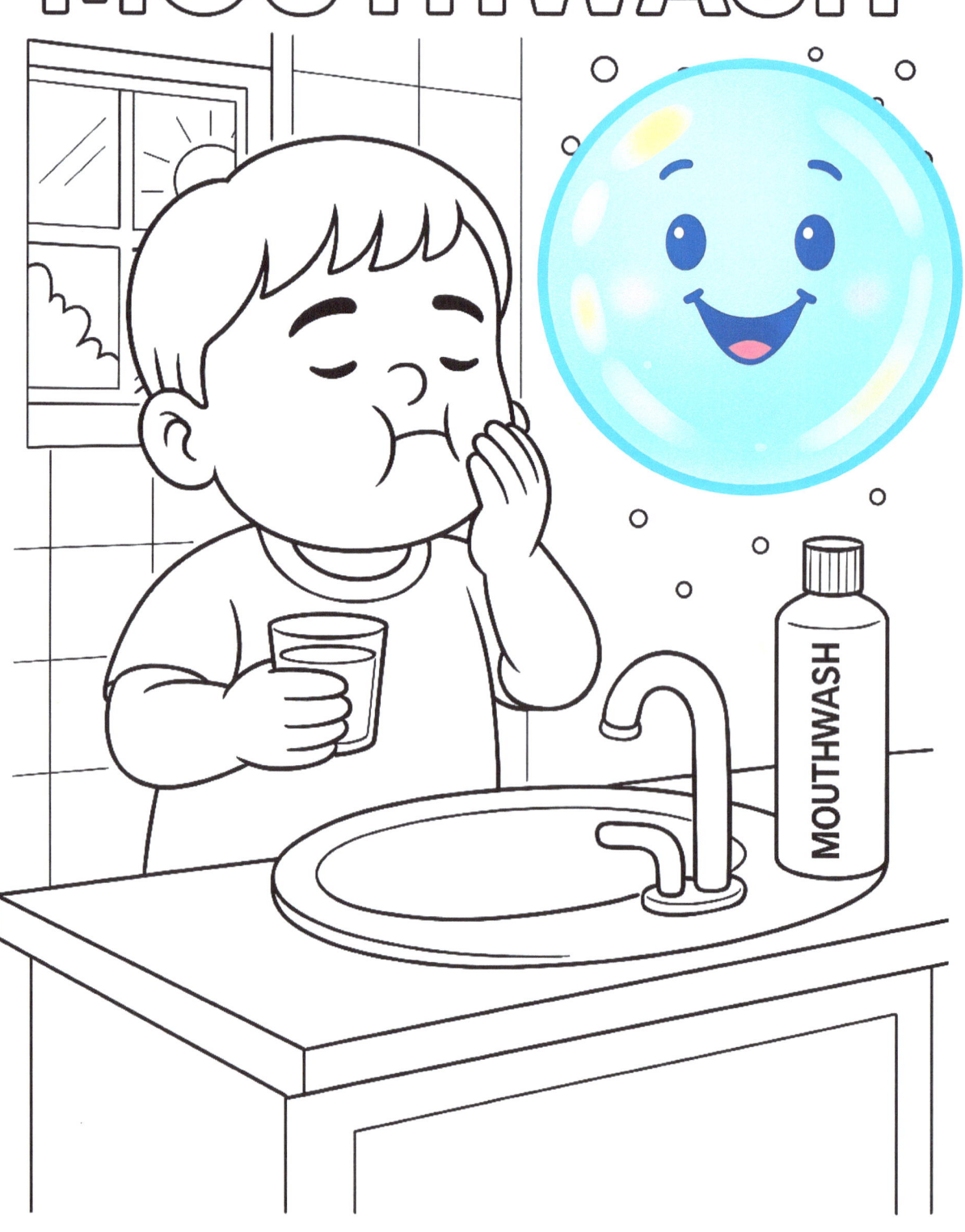

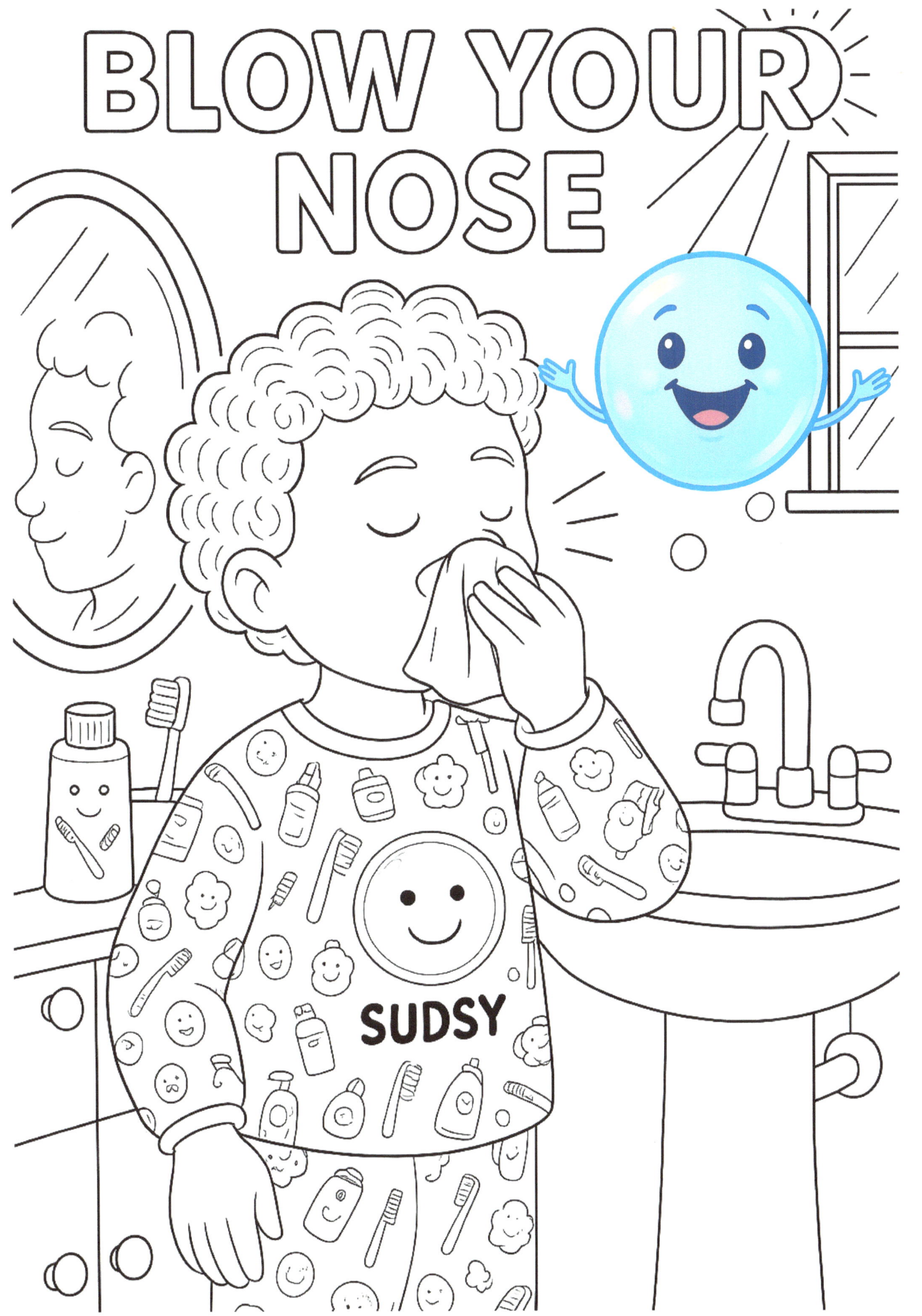

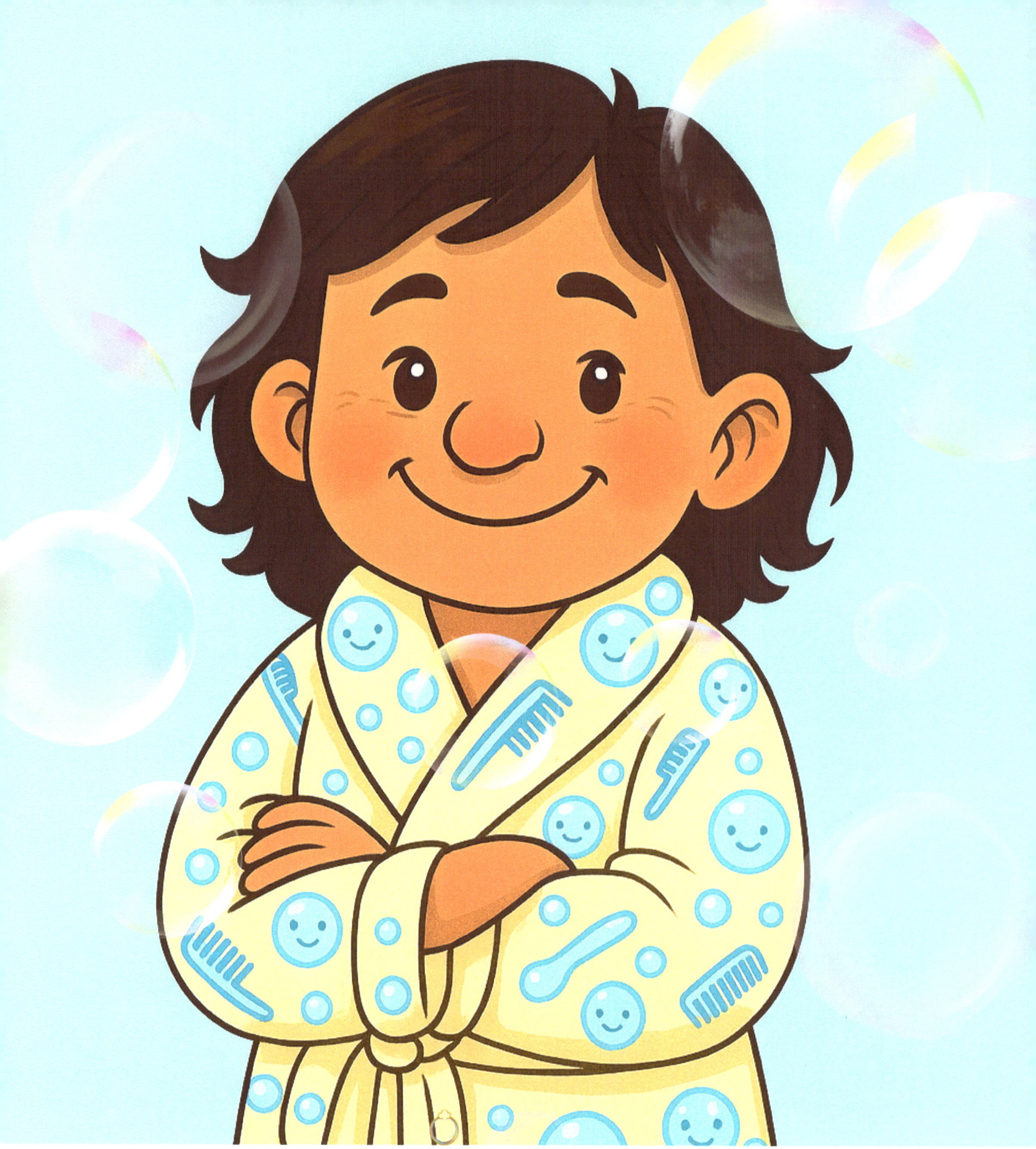

DRYING OFF & AFTERCARE

YOUR TOWEL ISN'T JUST FOR DRYING OFF

IT NEEDS CARE TOO!

REALLY GREAT TIPS

1. RINSE WASHCLOTH ONE FINAL TIME.

2. HANG CLOTH TO DRY ON A TOWEL RACK...

3. OR A SHAMPOO BOTTLE.

DAILY ROUTINE TIP!
YOU CAN USE A FRESH WASHCLOTH EVERY DAY OR YOU CAN REUSE THE SAME WASHCLOTH THE NEXT DAY FOR YOUR BOTTOM AREA ONLY. ALWAYS USE A CLEAN CLOTH FOR THE TOP OF YOUR BODY. REPEAT YOUR WASHING ROUTINE EVERY DAY!

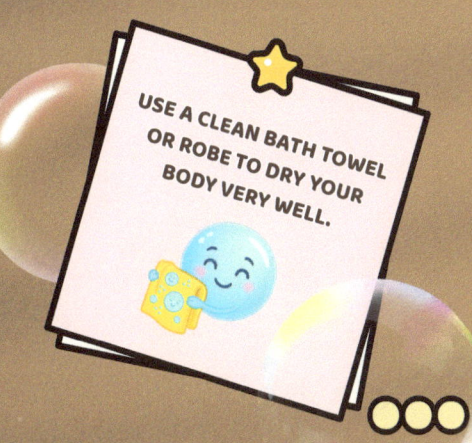

USE A CLEAN BATH TOWEL OR ROBE TO DRY YOUR BODY VERY WELL.

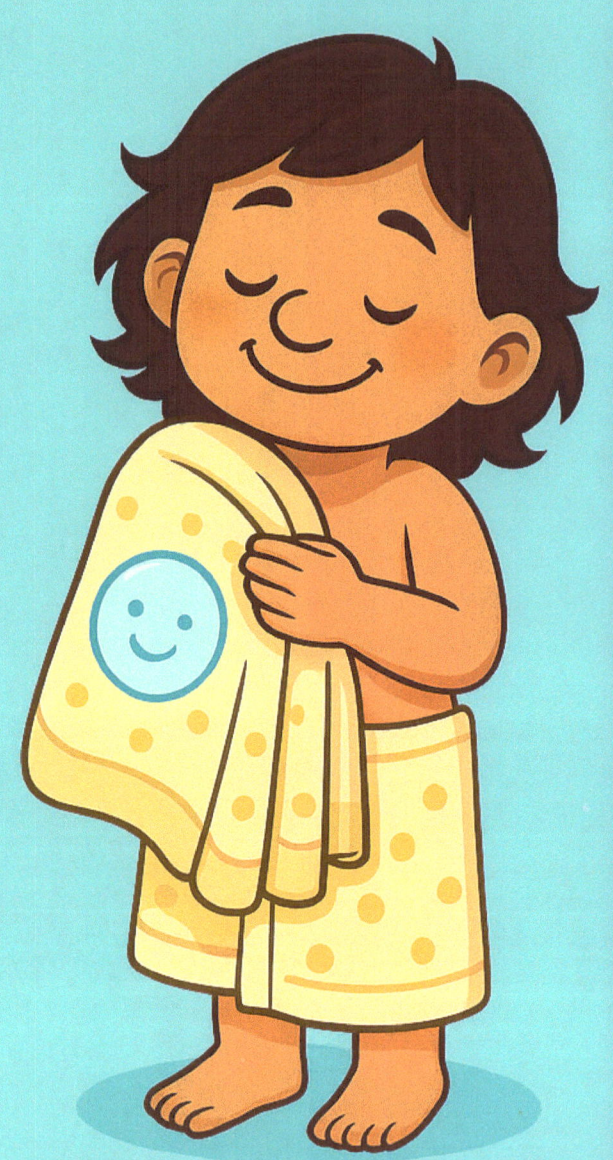
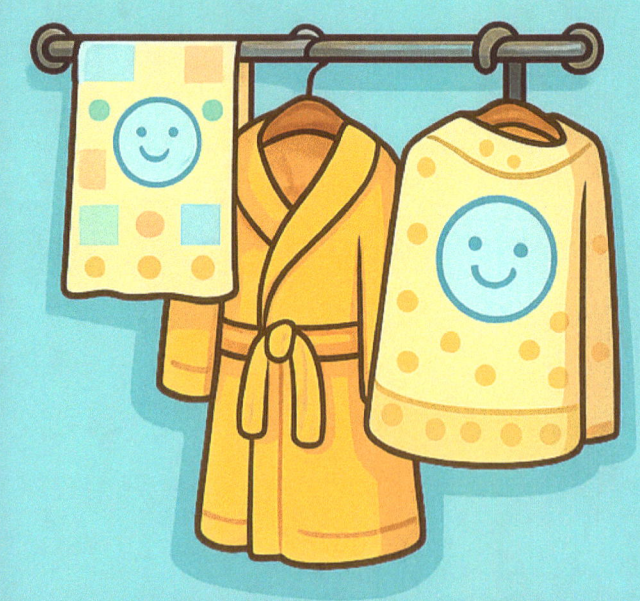
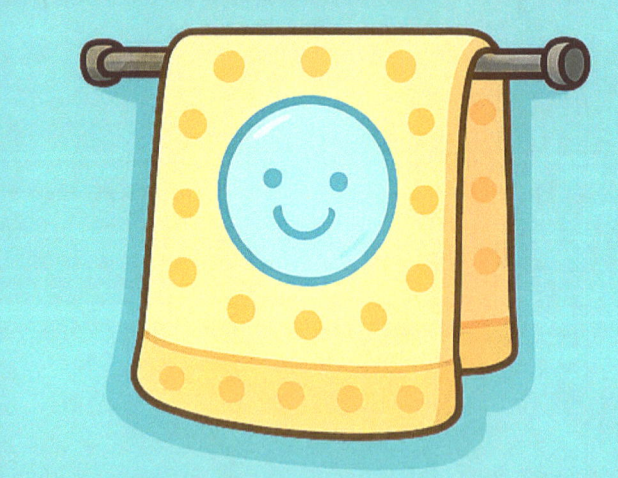

This helps keep germs and moisture away.
NEXT, APPLY A NICE MOISTURIZER OF YOUR CHOICE!
THIS INCLUDES:

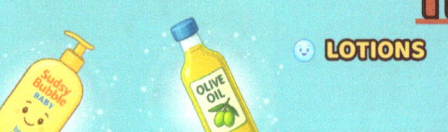

- LOTIONS
- OILS LIKE OLIVE, COCONUT OR BABY OIL
- BUTTERS, LIKE COCOA AND SHEA!

THESE HELP LOCK IN MOISTURE AND KEEP YOUR SKIN SMOOTH, SOFT AND HEALTHY!

AND IF YOU NEED IT, NOW'S THE TIME TO APPLY DEODORANT TO KEEP YOU NICE AND FRESH!

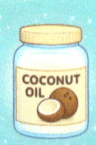
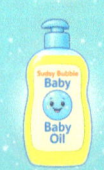
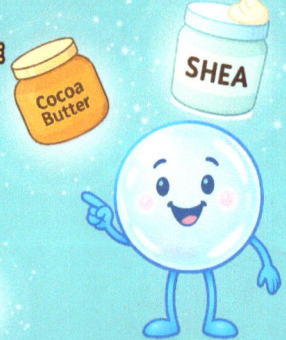

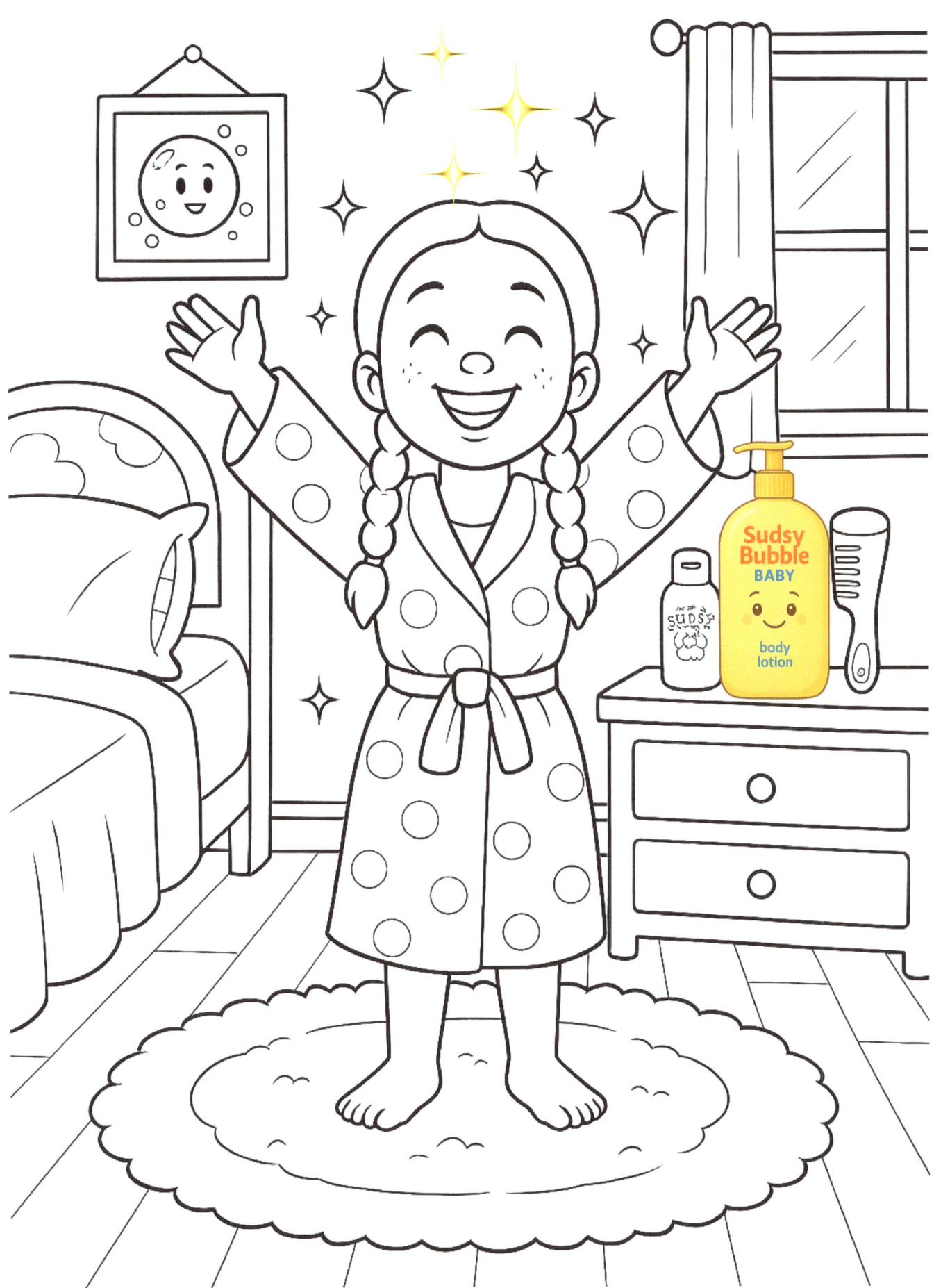

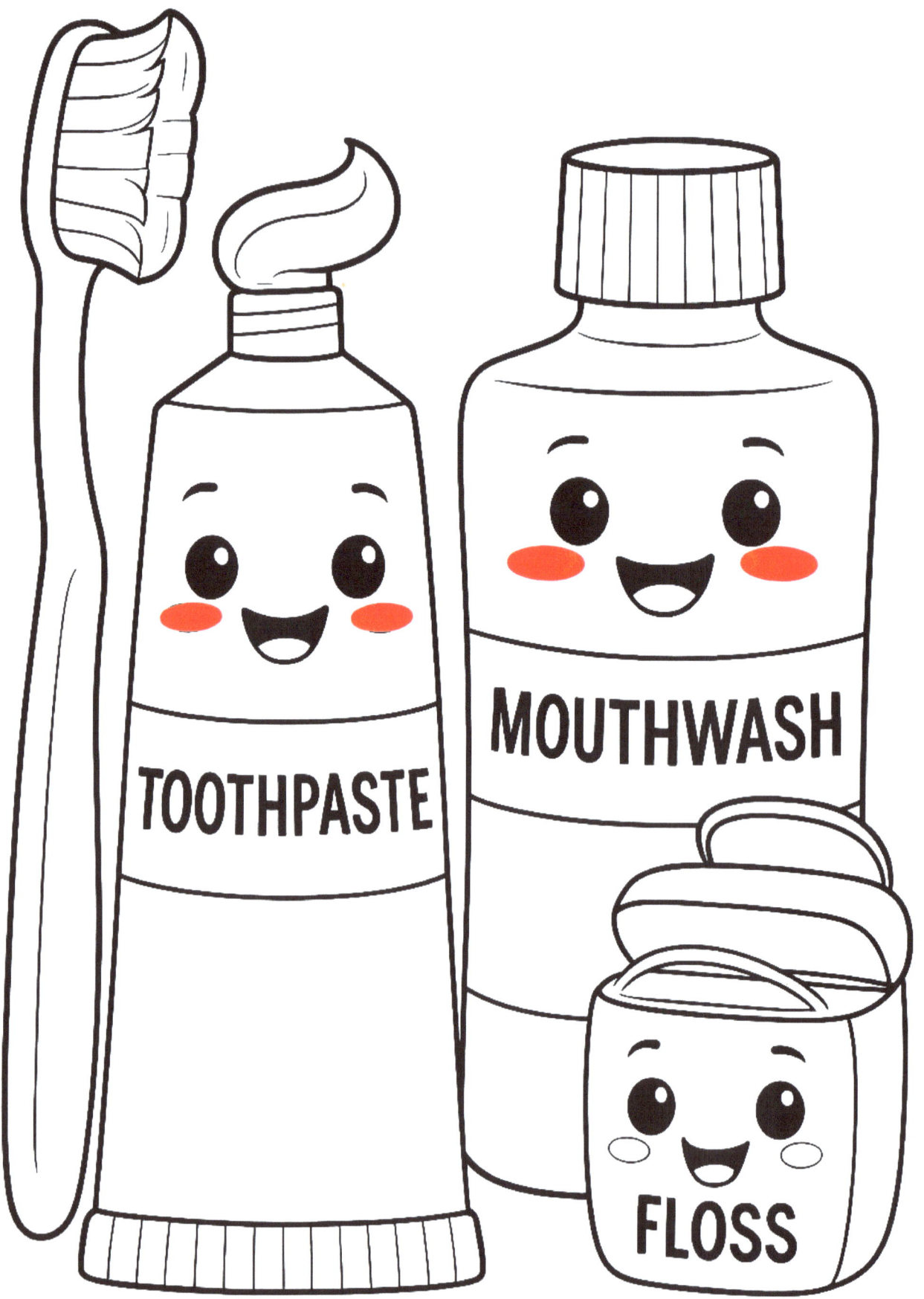

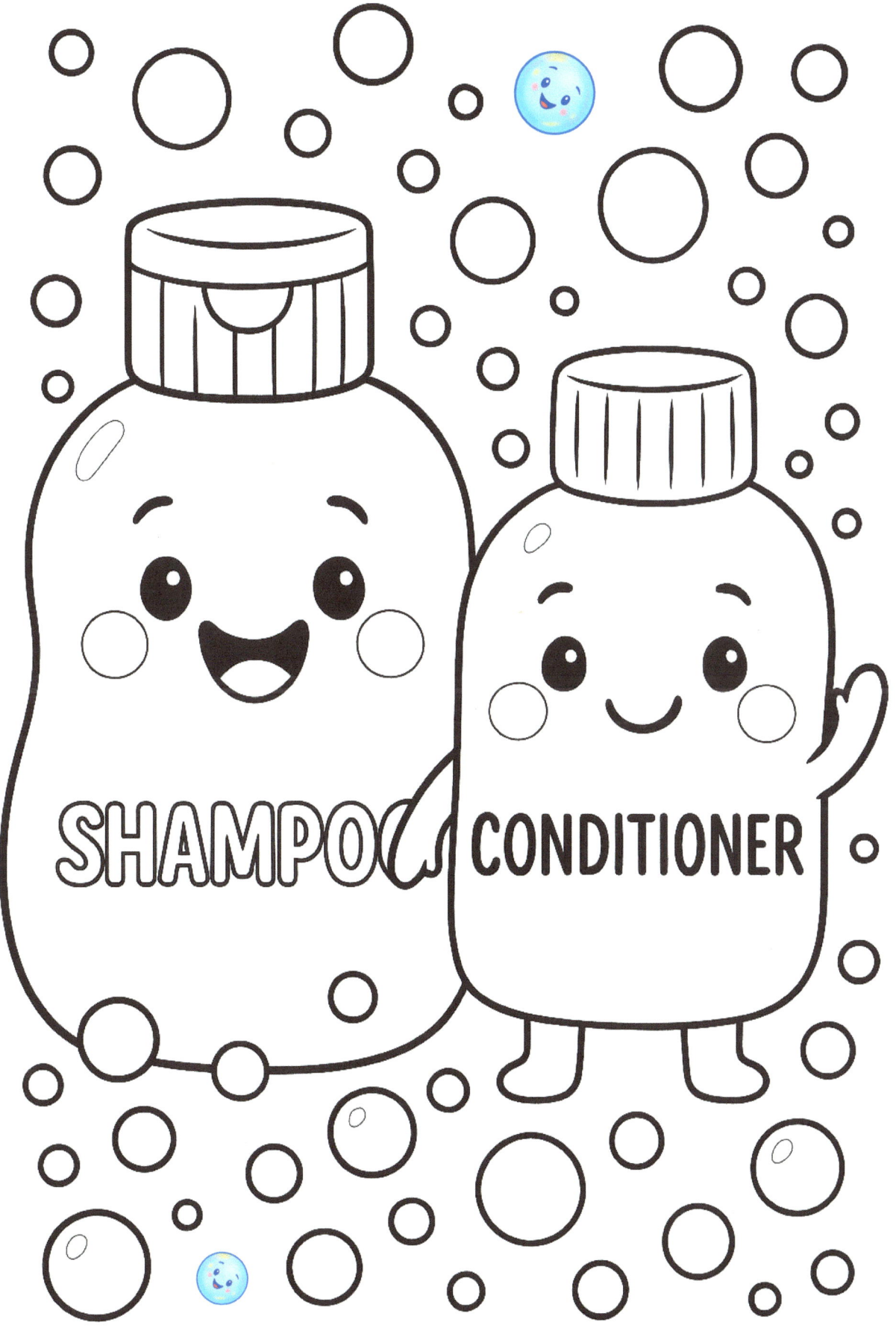

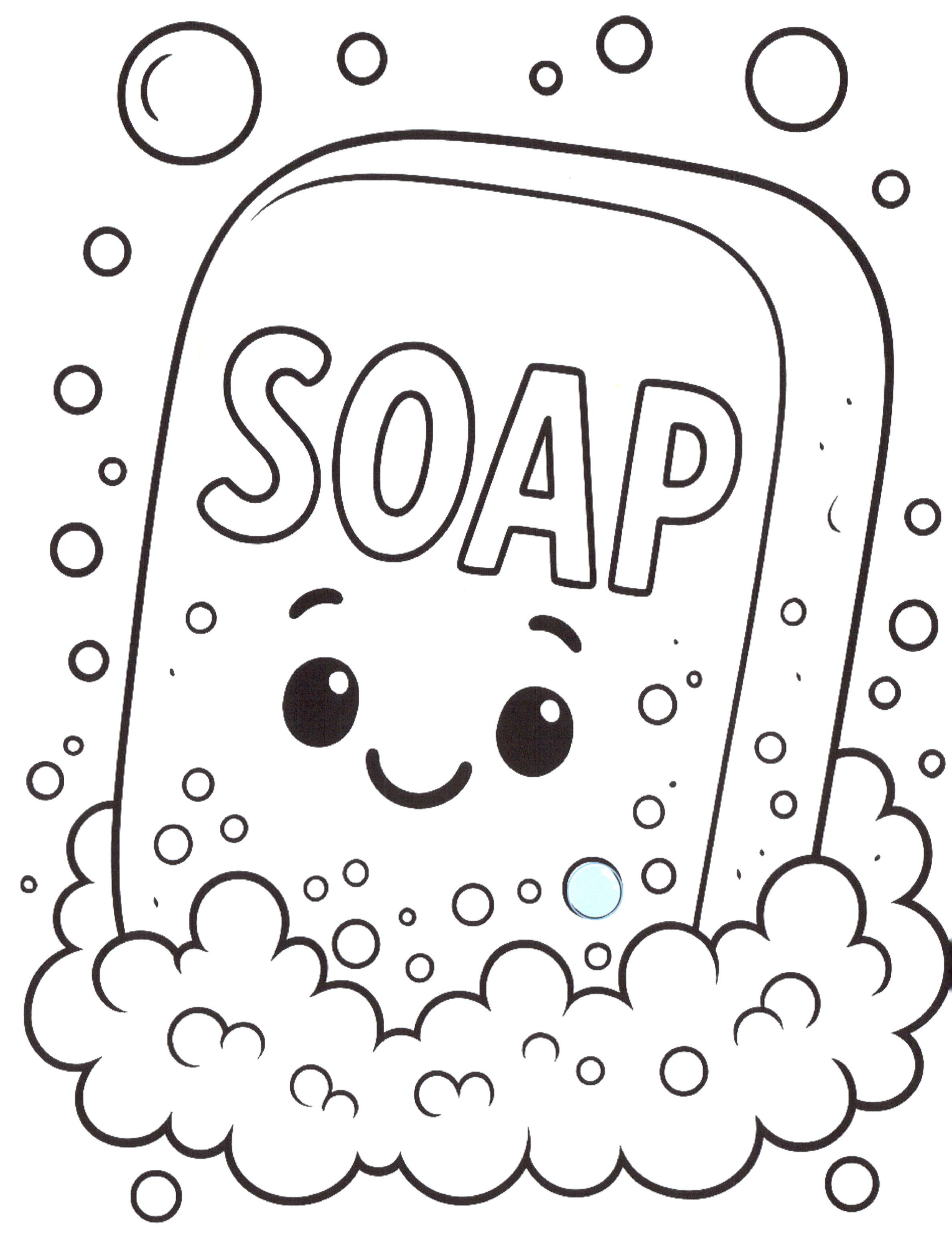

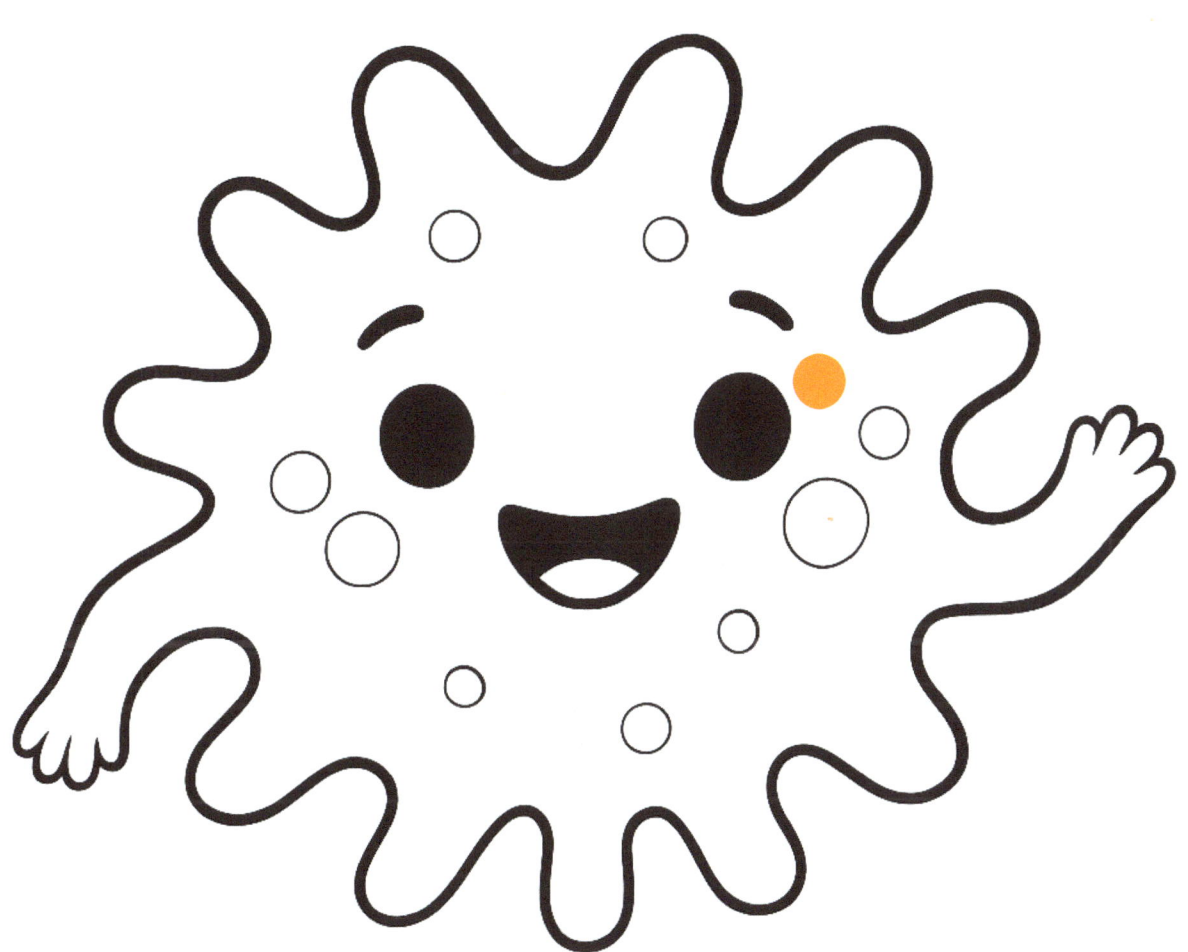

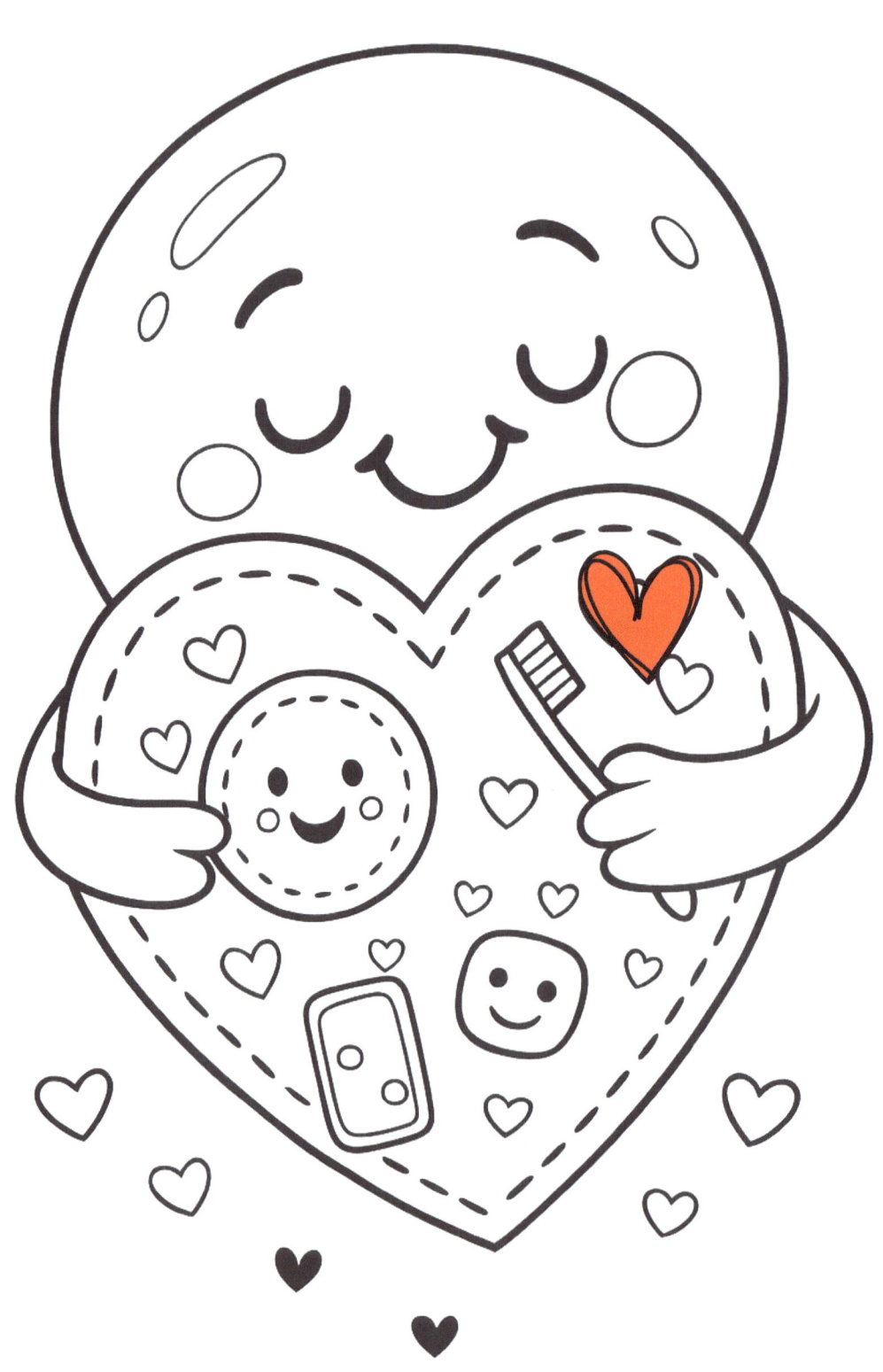

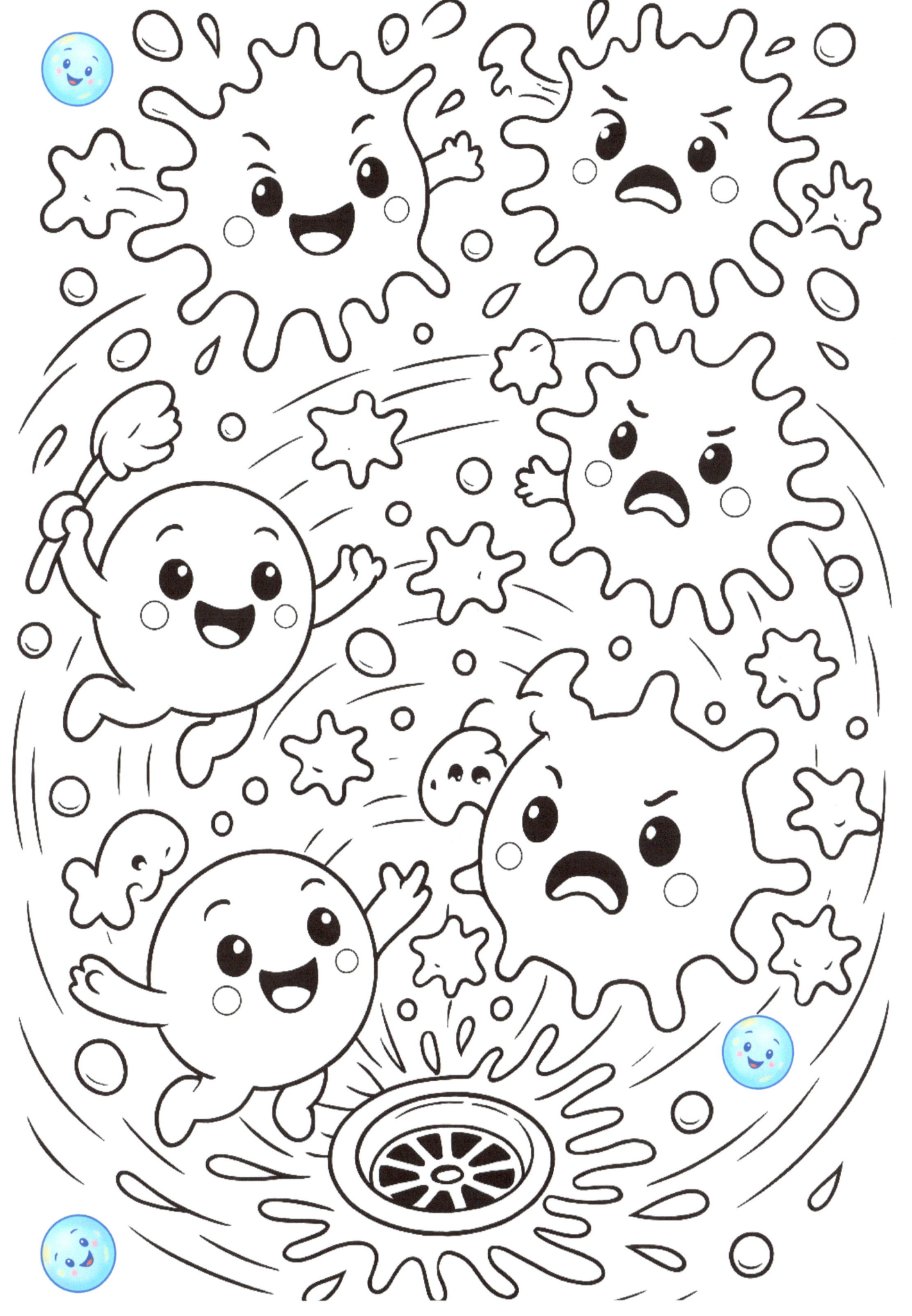

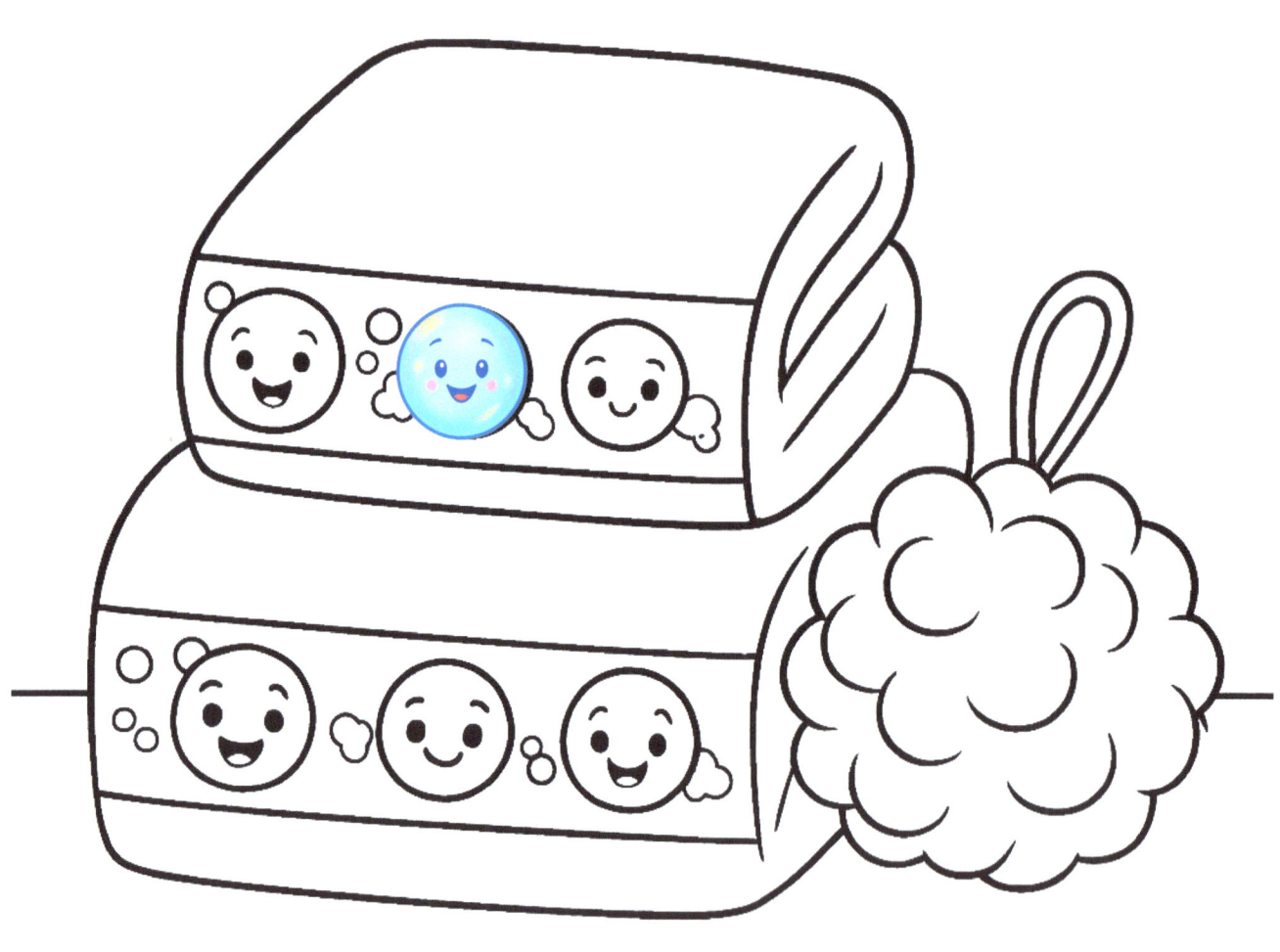

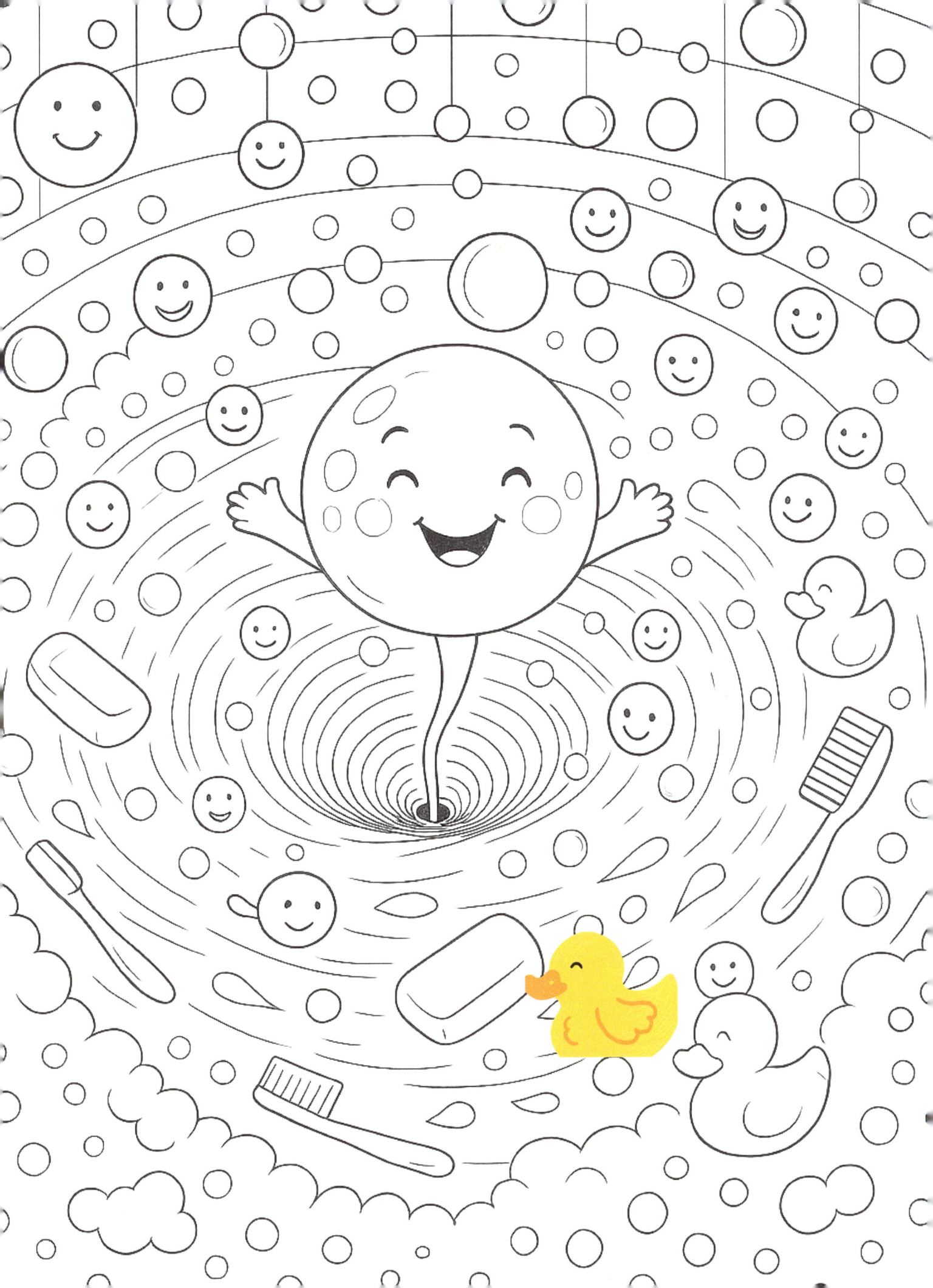

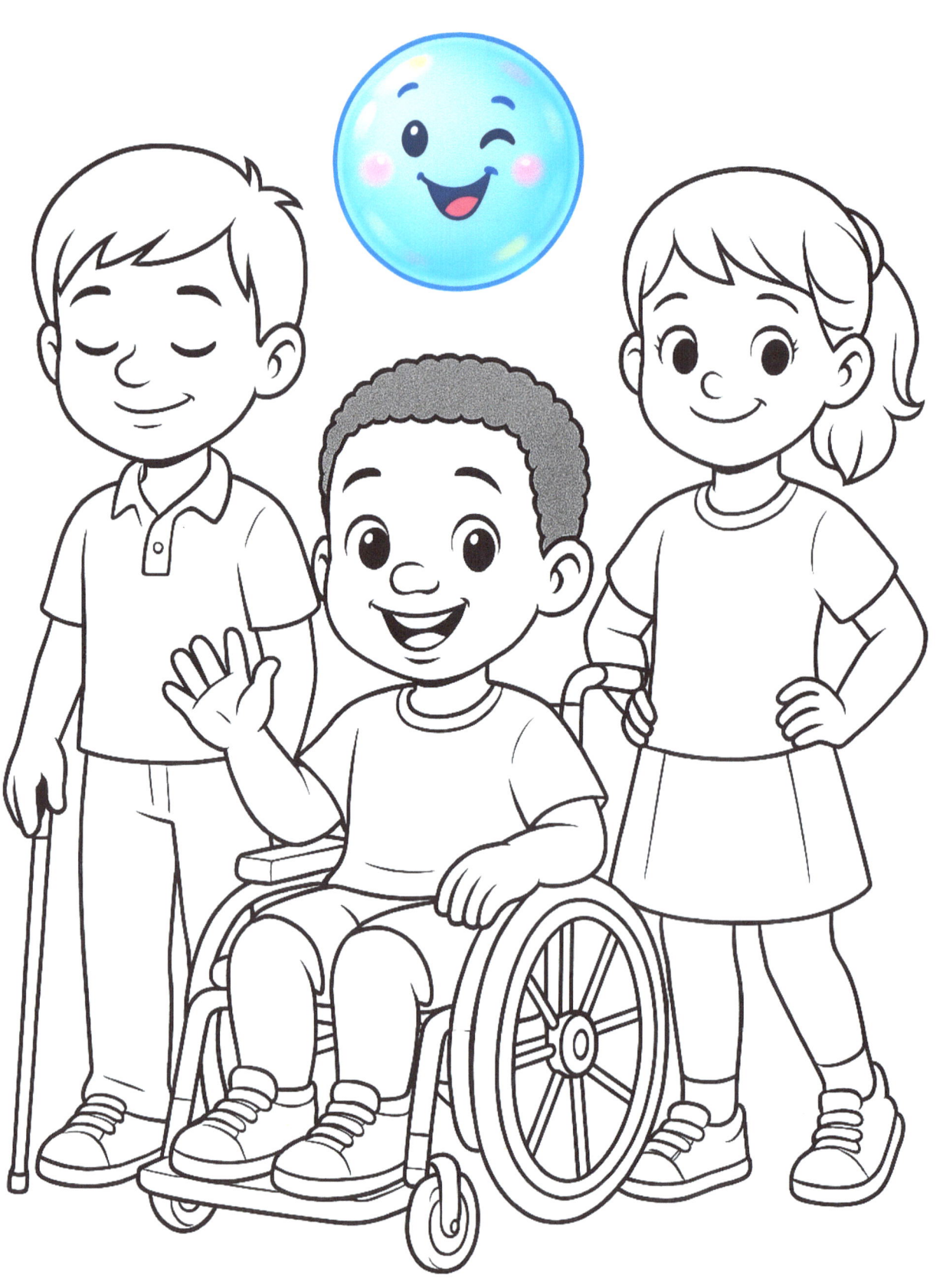

Wasn't that fun?!

Getting nice and clean with suds and bubbles always feels good! But guess what? Just like we clean the outside of our bodies, we must take care of the inside too. That's called internal hygiene and it's just as important...

1. We eat healthy foods and drink clean water to keep our bodies strong, but what about our minds and thoughts and feelings?

2. We take care of them by surrounding ourselves with happy, kind things. We take deep breaths and talk about our feelings when we're upset or anxious. And if we're okay with it, we can give and get big, tight hugs.

3. We also learn to notice when someone else is upset. Sometimes they might say or do things that aren't nice because they haven't learned to care for their feelings yet. This isn't your fault, and it's your right to protect your heart and mind from that, including walking away.

It's okay to say no
I love myself
I choose myself
I am enough
My feelings matter
It's okay to ask for help

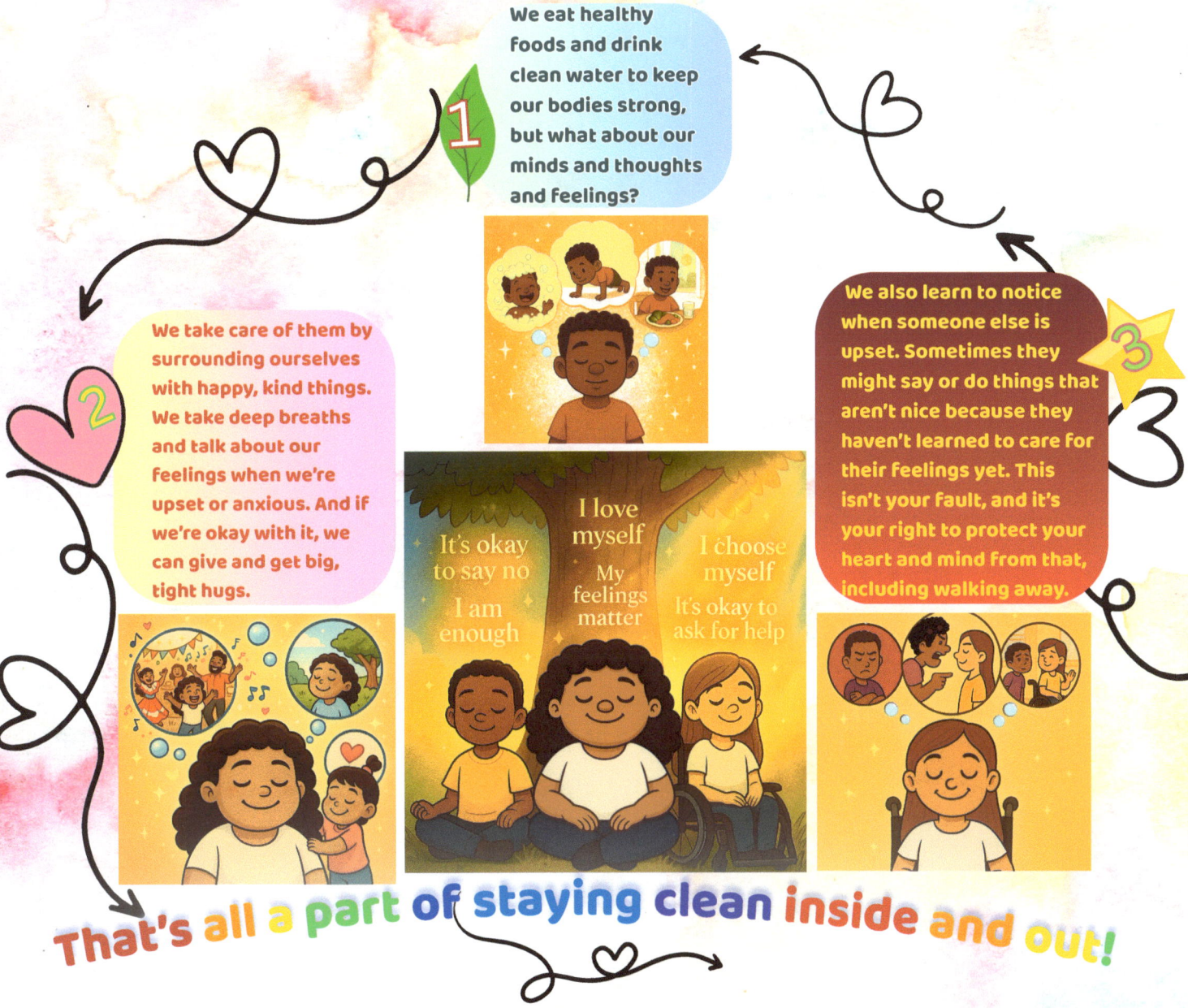

That's all a part of staying clean inside and out!

CARING FOR OUR HEARTS AND MINDS

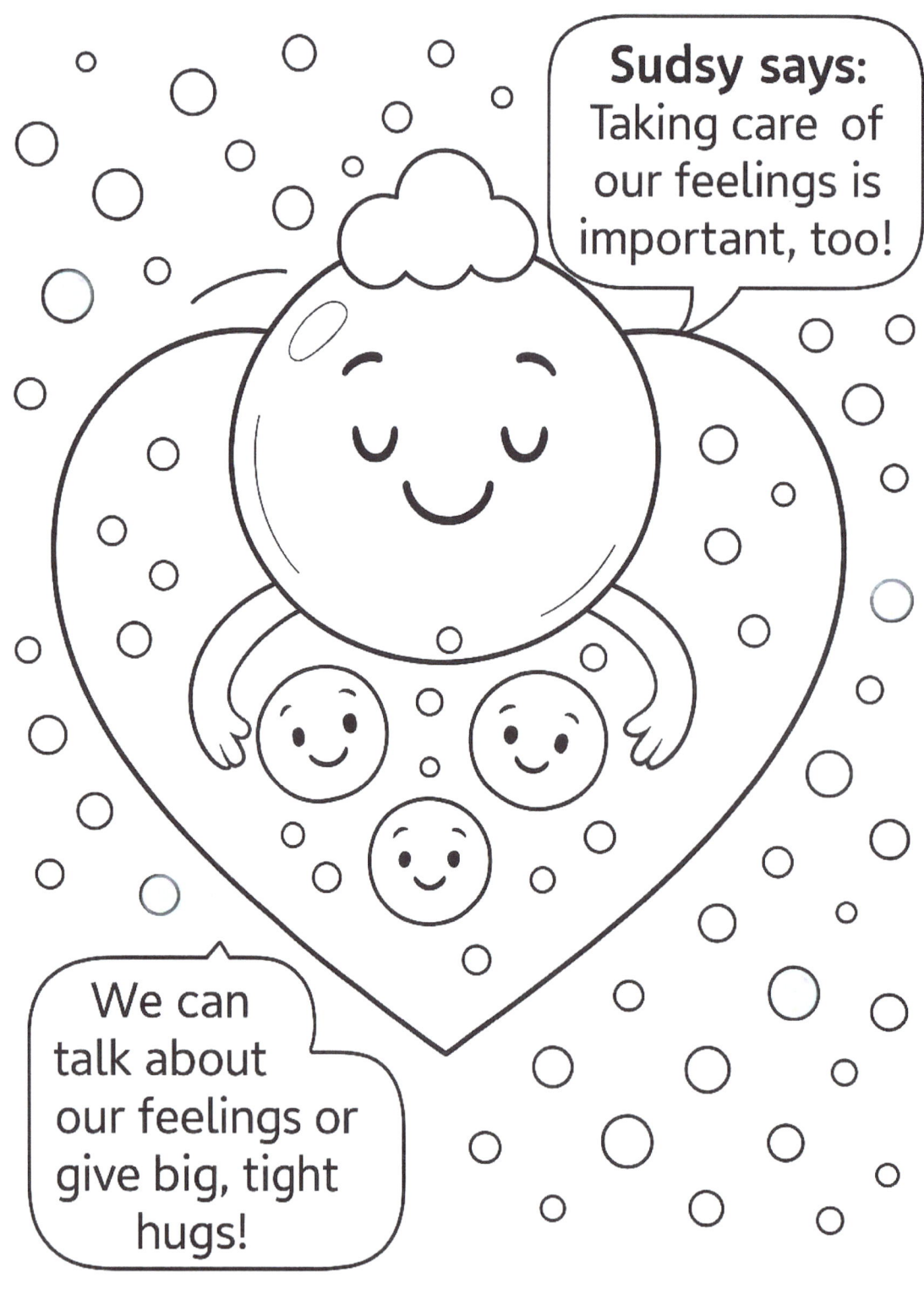

BEFORE YOU GO... LET'S RECAP!

1. Wash the night away, Wash the day away.
2. Wipe your bottom (front to back) before getting in the bath or shower with wipes or toilet paper until they stay white.
3. Wash your hair.
4. Wash your face.
5. Wash your upper body: chest, belly (DON'T FORGET YOUR BELLY BUTTON!), neck, arms, hands.

RINSE YOUR TOWEL & ADD FRESH SOAP

6. Wash your back.
7. Wash your underarms.

RINSE YOUR TOWEL & ADD FRESH SOAP

8. Wash your legs.

RINSE YOUR TOWEL & ADD FRESH SOAP

9. Wash your front, the creases of your legs and your bottom (front to back). Remember to wash and rinse EACH AREA two separate times.

RINSE YOUR TOWEL & ADD FRESH SOAP

10. Wash your feet top, bottom, between toes.
11. Check your fingernails. At this stage, they should be clean. If not, clean them with your nail brush or towel.
12. Final full body rinse.
13. Brush your teeth.
14. Moisturize your skin.
15. Hang your dry off towel and your washcloth to dry on a towel rack, hook or anywhere it can hang.
16. ALWAYS LOVE AND RESPECT YOURSELF!

Thank you for joining us today!

Remember, staying clean inside and out helps us feel good, look good, and be our best everyday! Me and the bubbies love you all just the way you are and can't wait to see you again very soon! Until next time friends!
Love,
Sudsy

www.ingramcontent.com/pod-product-compliance
Lightning Source LLC
Chambersburg PA
CBHW061156030426
42337CB00002B/23